PET ALLERGIES
Remedies for an Epidemic

by
Alfred J. Plechner, DVM
and
Martin Zucker

Foreword by William Shatner

DR. GOODPET LABORATORIES
VERY HEALTHY ENTERPRISES INC.
P.O. BOX 4489
INGLEWOOD, CA 90309

800-222-9932

Printed in the United States of America

First Edition

Library of Congress Catalogue Card Number 85-051341
ISBN 0-9615452-0-8

To the memories of
"Dune," "Paris," "Edson," "Alex" and "Ruppert,"
who gave me the inspiration to help other needy animals.

ABOUT THE AUTHORS

- **Dr. Alfred J. Plechner**, a 1966 graduate of the University of California–Davis School of Veterinary Medicine, practices in West Los Angeles. Over the years he developed a special interest in nutrition, allergy and the relationship of the endocrine system to small animal disease. His research and clinical observations on food-related disorders and endocrine-immune imbalances have been published in veterinary journals. He is a member of the American Animal Hospital Association, American Veterinary Medical Association, Southern California Veterinary Medical Association, and the Academy of Veterinary Allergy.

  Plechner has been interviewed on many TV and radio programs, including "Good Morning America" and "The Geraldo Show."

  He is co-creator of "Nature's Recipe" health food products for pets.

  Plechner maintains a wildlife refuge in the Santa Monica Mountains, providing free treatment for injured wild animals brought in by government agencies and concerned citizens. The facility is licensed by the U.S. Department of Interior Fish and Wildlife Service and the California State Department of Fish and Game. Proceeds from book sales are being used to help sustain and expand this unique treatment center.

- **Martin Zucker** is a free-lance writer who has been covering the health, nutrition and fitness field since 1975. He has authored a number of books, including three on nutrition and health-care for pets, and written many articles for national magazines. He is a contributing editor to "Let's Live Magazine" and "Men's Fitness Magazine." He has also spent many years studying natural health care.

TABLE OF CONTENTS

- **Acknowledgments**   VI
- **Foreword**   VII

- **Part One — The Epidemic**

1. *Roots Of An Epidemic*   3
2. *Is Pet Food Fit Food?*   11
3. *Food Allergies — Trouble By The Mouthful*   18
4. *Why Are Foods Allergenic?*   25
5. *Food Allergies Can Strike Anywhere*   33
6. *Missing Minerals*   40
7. *The Enzyme Connection*   48
8. *Breeder's Blight — The Genetic Problem*   52
9. *The Adrenal Timebomb*   60
10. *When The Timebomb Explodes (Dogs)*   69
11. *When The Timebomb Explodes (Cats)*   79
12. *Fleas, Insects And Inhalant Allergies*   85

- **Part Two — The Remedies**

13. *What — And What Not — To Do*   95
14. *The Hypoallergenic Diet*   97
15. *Mineral Supplementation*   102
16. *Topping Up The Enzymes*   104
17. *Hormonal Replacement Therapy*   106
18. *Prevention*   120
19. *Is There A Human Connection?*   125
20. *Pet Allergies Update*   127

- **Selected References**   131
- **Index**   133

ACKNOWLEDGMENTS

The authors would like to thank the following individuals for their contributions in the creation of this book:
- To the Miracle Mile art department staffers who applied their talents in bringing the book to print: Bill Lucas, Tevis Harvey, and Liz Castro.
- To Roz Wheelock, Jim Keel, Richard Wolters, and Suzanne Beedy, for sharing their special insight into the problems of breeding, and, for the second time, thanks to Persian breeder Laneen Firth for her candor and information.
- To Charlene Hunt and Judy Flerman, two favorite clients of mine, who helped me explain the serious problems afflicting many of the guide dogs for the blind.
- To Officer Jay Broyles of the Beverly Hills Police Department, for sharing the story of "Boss," the No. 1 police dog in the world.
- To Dr. Michael Fox of the Institute for the Study of Animal Problems.
- To Jim Murchison for technical advice, and Jeff Abel, of Overload Publications in Torrance, for extending courtesy in a time of need.

FOREWORD

(Actor William Shatner has been a Doberman Pinscher enthusiast for more than 30 years. "A dog in my life is as natural as kids or a car," he says. One of his dogs, named "Kirk" after the futuristic space captain he has made famous in the TV and cinema Star Trek series, placed second in its breed competition at Westminster, the country's most prestigious dog show.")

During the mid-1970s, "Heidi," one of my young Dobermans, was having great difficulties standing. It was "wobblers syndrome" and she would have to be put down, one vet said.

I went to Al Plechner for a second opinion. He looked at the x-rays and said it wasn't "wobblers." To my amazement, he said the problem was diet and that he thought he could improve "Heidi" merely by changing her food. I followed his recommendations, and in a couple of weeks the dog was much better. Soon she was perfectly normal again, and stayed that way, a very healthy dog, until she died at age 14.

"Heidi's" problem was, of all things, a beef allergy that severely affected her hind legs. Once beef was removed from her diet, she was fine.

I have been breeding Dobermans for many years and have watched with great alarm the genetic problems that are increasingly afflicting this breed — thin, falling hair, sores, dry coat, chronic cough.

The Dobies of the past were not the same genetically damaged animals as today's Dobies. The more inbred they have become, the more problems have surfaced. As you will see in this revealing book, a crisis in health and survival has developed that envelopes not just Dobermans, but many, many breeds of dogs and cats.

Al Plechner's innovative research into food, allergies and hormonal relationships has had a big impact on the health of my dogs. All of them, thanks to him, are doing just fine.

What Al practices, I believe, is the cutting edge of veterinary medicine. He is a concerned animal doctor who cares about animals, someone not content to merely treat the symptoms of diseases. He looks for their causes.

As the results of improper breeding become more and more evident in the growing incidence of disease, the work of dedicated people like Al Plechner becomes all that more important.

William Shatner
Los Angeles, March 1990

PART ONE

The Epidemic

1

Roots Of An Epidemic

Are your cats and dogs eternally scratching?
Are there ''hot spots'' of raw, red flesh on their bodies?
Is there loss of hair?
Severe reactions to flea-bites and ear mites?
Do your animals carry, or suffer from, potentially deadly viruses?
Do they suffer from frequent diarrhea?
Vomiting?
Weight loss?
Epileptic seizures?
Chronic liver disease?
Kidney ailments?
Hyperactivity?
Lethargy?
Do your animals simply have less good health than you think they should?
If they could talk, would they tell tales of woe like the following:

● ''Kahlua,'' a two-year-old Golden Retriever, enjoyed reasonably good health, marred perhaps by an occasional summer itchy skin. One day a friend advised her owners that she needed a higher protein diet. So the owners bought the most expensive commercial formulation on the market and fed it to ''Kahlua.'' Within eight hours, the dog developed a hive-like reaction over her body, followed by shaking, vomiting and diarrhea. The owners, thinking they had introduced the new food too fast, backed off and mixed smaller amounts of the new food in with the old. The same thing happened. The dog couldn't tolerate something in the new diet.

● ''Henry,'' a three-year-old domestic shorthair cat, was fed a predominantly beef diet by his owner since being obtained from a rescue organization. For a year there was no problem. The owner then decided to put some variety in the animal's diet and introduced canned tuna. Almost immediately, ''Henry'' began vomiting and his ears became inflamed and swollen.

● ''Buddy,'' a seven-year-old fox terrier, had been fed the same diet all his life. He was always a healthy animal but now had developed a terrible skin rash. He bit and chewed his feet. His ears became thick and swollen. A bald patch was spreading near his tail. The diagnosis was flea allergy reaction. But that wasn't all. He also had a history of chronic ear mites. Upon examination, "Buddy" was found to have a genetic defect causing profound endocrine-immune imbalances. He was hypersensitive to his food and environment.

● "Flower," a purebred Burmese, had an irresistable personality, but was very small and frail despite a ravenous appetite. She was plagued by a chronic sneeze, along with runny, red eyes, and inflamed gums that produced a bad odor. By age one she developed feline leukemia and soon died. She was a glamour kitty, the offspring of champions. But physically she was an endproduct, a defective cat programmed for an early death.

● "Nancy," a two-year-old Cocker Spaniel from a prominent line of champions, had been in and out of animal hospitals since her owners bought her as a young puppy. She gained weight very slowly, developed a chronic ear infection at 4 months, an itchy rash on the stomach shortly thereafter, and suffered from epileptic seizures. On occasion, she acted aggressively towards her human family. "Nancy" still hadn't come into heat. She suffered from a genetic adrenal deficiency seriously affecting her overall health and behavior.

THE UNRECOGNIZED EPIDEMIC

Acute or chronic, early in life or later, mixed breed or blueblood, the foregoing accounts all have a common denominator. In each scenario is an animal who has lost the ability to cope with the environment — with food, with viruses, with bacteria, with insects, with life. These animals have become sickly before their time.

They represent the tip of a massive, unchartered iceberg — an epidemic of disease — that is not yet fully recognized by the veterinary medical profession. At this very time, millions of our domestic pets are going down, like the Titanic, and will continue to do so unless we take steps to avert what I consider is a very real and growing disaster.

The problem is two-fold:

1) Over the last thirty or forty years there has been a proliferation of improperly designed commercial pet food. It is typically filled with poor-quality ingredients and chemical additives and bears little resemblance to food created by Mother Nature. Minimum daily nutritional requirements may be met by some products but they are just that — minimums. Many products don't even meet minimum standards. Manufacturers often put more effort into cosmetic effects for you, the buyer, than into nutritional quality for the animal. They want food that looks good to eat. Whether it is good enough for the animal to live on is another matter. Among pets there is widespread intolerance of commercial foods. This rejectivity shows up as violent sickness or chronic health problems. It often triggers a hypersen-

sitivity and overreaction to flea and insect bites, pollens, soaps, sprays and environmental contaminants.

2) Similarly, over the last fifty years or more, intensive breeding for particular physical features has created seriously defective animals with impaired ability to tolerate their environments. These purebred cats and dogs may have the fashionable features valued by fanciers and judges, but the cost is high: animals with inferior equipment for survival, for health. Such animals enter life less able to cope and begin to have problems early on. And not only are biological flaws passed on to purebred offspring but to mixed breed descendants as well.

These two elements — poor food and genetic defects — have created an allergy disease epidemic ravaging our pet population.

An allergy is defined by medical dictionaries as "a hypersensitive state acquired through exposure to a particular allergen." An allergen is any agent that can bring out an immediate or delayed reaction.

Based on twenty years in practice, I think the meaning of allergy as it pertains to veterinary medicine should read something like this: A hypersensitive state either inherited or acquired that is ruining the health of millions of pets and seriously threatening their survival.

Strong stuff? Well, I don't say it lightly. On a daily basis in my practice I see cats and dogs by the numbers, with inferior or damaged immunity, who are seriously affected by environmental input. The experts really don't know the extent of allergies among pets. Some say 5-10 percent. Guestimates for food allergies alone begin at 1 and range all the way up to 30 percent.

I think the problem is much bigger, greater than anybody realizes. I think perhaps one out of two animals brought in to veterinary hospitals today may be suffering from some degree of allergic malady, a hypersensitive state that can cause death just as easily as it can cause an everyday scratching problem. Allergies are so common that pet owners probably face the problem sometime or another during the lifespan of their animals.

I have seen unmistakable patterns of disease poking pathetically out of kingly breeding lines and unmistakable patterns of sickness resulting from consumption of specific diets. Long ago I said, "Whoa, Plechner, something's going on here." And I began my detective work. I began looking for causes.

CAUSE NO. 1: FLAWED FOOD

Within five years in practice, I became aware that many of the cats and dogs brought in for treatment seemed to have some sort of hypersensitivity condition such as itchy skin, red mucousy eyes, or overreaction to flea bites. It was so common I began to wonder if I had missed the boat in school. I didn't remember any academic fuss — any emphasis at all — about allergies. I never had the remotest expectation I would be seeing this so frequently. Was I seeing what I was seeing? Or just seeing things?

I was going by the book, using the standard treatments that all veterinarians used. I did what I had been taught to do. And I reviewed my textbooks and journals to make sure I was on track. I did skin scrapings. Skin biopsies. Intradermal allergy testing for 175 different allergens. Desensitizing programs. I took blood samples. I used cortisone to stop inflammation. I dispensed the recommended pills, shots, soaps, ointments and powders.

But results were mixed. Nothing seemed to work consistently. Animals would often benefit temporarily but the signs would come marching back.

I purchased whatever was available in professional literature and took continuing education courses. But they provided little help and no inspired direction for inquiry or treatment. However, the new information did confirm the validity of my diagnoses. I was indeed seeing an extremely high number of animals with hypersensitivity, with allergic-like reactions.

I examined all the possibilities for allergy. There are only so many ways that allergens can enter the body and cause a reaction — through bites, fleas, contact directly through the feet and skin, through inhaling, and through eating.

In time I realized that many cases — with surprisingly widespread clinical signs — related directly to food. I wasn't seeing just the usual scratching or skin rashes or gastro-intestinal reactions you would expect from allergy, but things like epilepsy, liver and kidney ailments and other serious disease processes. There was a huge spectrum of conditions that didn't fit the mold of problems related to just allergy or just food. Eventually I was even able to determine how certain foods could affect certain areas on an animal's body.

I set out to design some dietary strategies that would enable pet owners to deal with the problem of food. To my amazement I found that about 30 percent of all the animals I was treating improved partially or wholly on modified diets in which certain antagonistic foods were eliminated.

With further sleuthing I discovered that many commercial food formulations are woefully deficient in key nutrients. This deficiency is a result of the abused state of the soil in which many of our agricultural crops are grown. I found that absence or insufficiency of important nutrients can also contribute to hypersensitivity. I also found that some vitamins — whether added to foods by the manufacturer or given to pets by their owners — can themselves cause allergic reactions.

My clinical research turned up still another major health clue related to food: many animals have enzyme deficiencies and are not able to properly process their food. This handicap creates nutritional deficiencies leading to allergic-like reactions and disease.

Altogether I determined that about half of the animals I was treating had problems related specifically to food and digestion. I also determined how they could be helped.

CAUSE NO. 2: THE GENETIC TIMEBOMB

The recent history of cosmetic breeding practices among cat and dog breeders is replete with bad news — animals with gross deformities, lost instincts, altered and bizarre behavior, and specific health problems. In many cases, the headlong rush for ribbons, cups, titles. prestige and sales results in highly defective animals.

Long ago I began to observe patterns of similar disease and allergy signs along breeding lines. Often these signs or reactions could be neutralized only through the use of cortisone, a drug commonly used by physicians and veterinarians. It acts as an anti-inflammatory agent and also reduces reaction to allergens. The drug is a synthetic and limited version of a highly protective and regulating hormone produced by the adrenal glands.

The parade of sick animals in my clinic raised two nagging questions:

1) In addition to well-documented genetic problems, could widespread cosmetic-oriented breeding also be producing hormonally-defective animals unable to adequately defend themselves against allergens, microorganisms and disease?

2) And could we, the veterinarians, unaware of the depth of such a possible genetic flaw, inadvertently be compensating for that deficiency while patching the surface signs with our massive use of cortisone drugs?

Years of clinical investigation gave me the answers — yes on both counts.

Yes, I was seeing a genuine genetic problem — an adrenal timebomb that sooner or later explodes inside many animals. Man, that most amateur of creators, was creating still more damage in the arrogant attempt to improve on God's own design.

In some cases, the timebomb goes off with a great bang. I've seen sobbing children carrying in the casualties — helpless pathetic animals, sometimes with oozing sores over their body, sometimes hairless and emaciated, sometimes so weak they can't stand, sometimes all of these.

The timebomb can also tick relentlessly for years, producing small problem after small problem that eventually develop into serious disease and organ failure.

In my opinion, it's a dinosaur effect. Animals are being programmed for disaster, for extinction. Many of them are biochemical cripples with defective adrenal glands unable to manufacture adequate cortisol, a hormone vital for health and resistance to disease.

The signs of this defect are expressed as various diseases which we veterinarians often treat with steroid drugs. There is generally strong reservation to use these drugs over a long period of time for fear of side effects. However, with the proper testing and the proper hormonal replacement, many severely allergic and sick animals can be restored back to health without suffering any side effects whatsoever. I have discovered, in fact, that if these deficient animals do not receive this kind of therapy — and often they need it for a lifetime — they will never get well. It's a new and powerful approach to serious disease.

HOW TO USE THIS BOOK

If you are an owner of purebreeds you may be asking yourself whether you have a timebomb on your hands. Is it ready to go off? Has it already gone off? What can you do to defuse the bomb and what can you do to minimize the damage if it has already gone off?

If you are the owner of mixed breeds don't think you've been spared. Many mixed animals carry the blood of champions within them. And that pure blood fraction may well contain the timebomb, the same defective genetic imprint. When animals breed naturally, according to their own choices, hybrid vigor makes for tough, resilient creatures. To what degree is the purebreed defect being perpetuated and elbowing out the hybrid vigor in your animals? What can you do about the timebomb in your mixed breed animals?

This book takes a piercing look at all the questions raised on these pages. It examines the role of food and neglected biochemical imbalances that together are creating an epidemic of allergy and disease among our pets. When recognized and understood they provide a powerful tool for dealing with health problems that otherwise may escape our best efforts to prevent and treat.

Most importantly, the book offers practical advice — remedies for the epidemic.

The solutions I propose are based on years of searching for alternatives to standard therapies that just don't work, or just work temporarily. These have been years of clinical research and trial and error — lots of trials, lots of errors and lots of failures, I should say. Happily, the long process led me to exciting treatment breakthroughs.

The ideas presented here have been effective for thousands of animals — perhaps over 8,000 of them by now — and they can certainly work for yours. I have crystallized my findings into an easy-to-follow, step-by-step plan which includes doing things both on your own and with the help of your veterinarian.

The basic problems I am concerned about are correctable and controllable. Even such deadly diseases as feline leukemia and feline infectious peritonitis can be better managed by following my guidelines.

The book is divided in two parts. The first covers the following problems, many of them overlooked in general veterinary medicine, that can severely impact the health of animals:

● The food connection, providing startling details about how commercial pet food can undermine animal health.

● Food allergies, a frequent source of irritation and upset and cause of both acute and chronic illness.

 ● My "Allergic HIT List" of major food offenders and the surprising scope of health problems they can cause.

 ● Mineral deficiencies, the depleted state of pet food, reflecting the depleted state of American agricultural soil.

 ● Enzyme deficiencies, a usually undiagnosed cause of ailments.

 ● How fad breeding practices have caused a multiplicity of serious genetic health problems.

 ● One such overlooked problem — the devastating adrenal deficiency.

 ● How animals are made super-sensitive to flea, insect and environmental allergies.

Part two contains the plan of action — using combinations of hypoallergenic diets, mineral and enzyme supplementation, and hormonal replacements. In my practice I find I can help about fifty percent of the sick animals with diet and supplements. When that doesn't work, I test for hormonal imbalances, prescribe the appropriate replacements and am able to successfully treat and provide lasting relief for a large percentage of the most resistant cases.

I will tell you how to apply these measures — some of them on your own, some through your veterinarian.

In Chapter Seventeen, I have compiled comprehensive testing and hormonal replacement details for veterinarians. This is the first time such information appears in a book. Among other things, it explains why long-term cortisone therapy is necessary in many cases and how it can be safely administered with maximum health benefits.

I am a big believer in prevention. So I will have an important chapter packed with practical information on how to avoid problems.

My goal in writing this book is to show you how to prevent health problems in the first place and if your animals do have problems then to explain how best to deal with them in the most effective way possible.

Many stubborn conditions can be remedied, just as in the following cases:

 ● "Silky," a one-year-old Doberman at the time, was brought in for a second opinion. His condition had been diagnosed as ulcerative colitis, a serious intestinal disorder, and it was recommended he be put to sleep. He had chronic diarrhea and was literally starving to death. We determined the dog to be suffering from a straightforward food allergy — beef and chicken, among other things — and we put him on a non-meat hypoallergenic diet. The dog recovered and today is a beautiful specimen.

 ● "Big Foot," a two-year-old grey tabby, had a classical case of feline infectious peritonitis. He had the typical distended abdomen filled with fluid. Blood tests revealed a cortisol problem. We initiated the appropriate hormone replacements. In three months the cat shed the virus and eventually regained full health.

 ● "Samantha," a three-year-old domestic shorthair, suffered from weight loss and anemia associated with feline leukemia. We determined the presence of the genetic biochemical insufficiency along with a sensitivity to beef and tuna. We prescribed a treatment program that addressed both problems. The cat fully recovered and tested negative for leukemia.

These were animals who normally would have been put to sleep. Today they are all thriving. Read on to see how you can remedy similar problems...or better yet, prevent them.

2

Is Pet Food Fit Food?

More than 30 percent of the ailments I treat in my practice are directly related to food. After reading this chapter I think you'll understand why that's so.

Next time you are stocking up on pet food at your favorite pet store or supermarket, step back and take a good look at the lineup of cans, packages and sacks in front of you.

What you see is mega-business — sales of $5 billion dollars a year. Americans spend four times more on pet food than on baby food, and twice as much than on cereal, macaroni, and flour products. In 1973, pet foods overtook coffee as the largest-selling category among dry grocery commodities.

Competition is fierce among the several thousand manufacturers. They spend more than $160 million a year on TV, newspaper and magazine advertising. They broadside you with trick photography, meaningless and misleading nutritional claims, and tongue-tickling names such as "Meow Mix," "Fish Ahoy," "Snausages," "Lollipups" and "Doggie Donuts."

In the competitive scramble, quality and good nutrition are often sacrificed to economics and profit. There are no government standards regulating quality. Quality is like shifting sands. It changes even within single product lines of a company as cheaper ingredients are constantly sought to replace more expensive ones.

Most people want to feed their pets cheaply and conveniently. So price is always an overriding commercial consideration.

One manufacturer concerned about nutritional quality in the industry summed up in print what we veterinarians have known for years: food is the cause of many routinely diagnosed ailments.

"There is one major reason that considerable tonnage of pet food is nutritionally inadequate, and that is competition," wrote Robert Pett of Pett Food Company in the March 1985 issue of DVM, a veterinary journal. "On one end of the battle line is price, causing the use of cheap ingredients, and on the other is the quest to enhance appeal through the use of chemicals."

Feeding cheaply can cost more in the long run — in veterinary bills.

In 1983, the University of California-Davis alerted veterinarians to be on the lookout for a potentially-serious skin disease traced to consumption of various generic dry dog foods sold in supermarket chains.

Dr. Anna Clark, the veterinary columnist for the Los Angeles Times, commented that many veterinarians and dog breeders are familiar with these cheaper generic foods and call them "starvation diets."

"Probably not all generic pet foods provide inadequate diets, but it would appear that, overall, the old you-get-what-you-pay-for adage applies here," she said.

But even expensive high-profile brands come a cropper now and then as they attempt to cut corners. Recently, a top specialty diet was found responsible for the deaths of highly-trained working dogs. The investigation revealed that the company had been using peanut shells for fiber in the product. Unfortunately, one lot of shells were contaminated with fungus that produced a lethal toxin.

Peanut shells?

Uh huh. They're cheap and add volume to the product.

FEATHERS, BEAKS, HOOVES, HORNS AND DISEASED TISSUE

Manufacturers are highly creative in concocting penny-pinching recipes. James Corbin, a professor of animal science at the University of Illinois, once cited some of the more unheralded ingredients used in cheap canned foods. The list included "gristle, hair, lungs, pig feet, pig snouts, tails, cheeks, udders, and condemned hog livers."

Condemned parts and animals rejected for human consumption are routinely re-routed for commercial pet foods. A similar fate applies to so-called 4-D animals. These are feed animals picked up dead, or that are dying, diseased, or disabled, and do not meet human-food qualifications. They are processed straightaway for pet consumption. Little goes to waste.

Food processing refuse of all sorts winds up in your animals' dinner bowls. Moldy grains. Rancid foods. Meat meal. The latter is ground-up slaughterhouse discards often containing disease-ridden tissue and high levels of hormones and pesticides — the very things that may have contributed to the death of the steer or hog.

In the book "Dr. Pitcairn's Complete Guide to Natural Health for Dogs and Cats," Dr. P.F. McGargle is quoted as saying that feeding such slaughterhouse wastes to pets "increases their chances of getting cancer and other degenerative diseases."

From his experience as a veterinarian and a federal meat inspector, McGargle says that these products "can include moldy, rancid or spoiled processed meats, as well as tissues too severely riddled with cancer to be eaten by people."

You commonly see the word byproducts on pet food ingredient lists. Do you know what it means? Euphemistically speaking, byproducts imply discards, rejected matter, fecal matter, and parts guaranteed not to make your mouth water.

Chicken byproducts include feathers, beaks, feet, waste material, the leftover parts after poultry has been slaughtered and processed for human consumption.

Beef byproducts include hooves, horns, skin with hair, esophagus, leftover organs and glands.

Who would buy a product if such contents were disclosed? Byproducts is clearly an alias designed to cover up the truth. Usually byproducts are high up on the ingredient list, meaning they comprise a good chunk of the contents. Byproducts often make up a big part of the total protein. Your animals utilize such ingredients poorly, if at all.

The diseased tissue, pus, hair, assorted slaughterhouse rejects, and carcasses in varying states of decomposition are sterilized with chemical, heat, and pressure procedures. Then crafty processing techniques are applied to fashion a "food" that tastes and looks good. Finally, product labels are written by shrewd merchandisers who hide more than they tell.

In 1983, the Pet Food Institute, representing the pet food industry, successfully petitioned the Food and Drug Administration for changes in labeling information. These proposals were made: "cheese" to describe cheese rinds, "vegetable fiber" to describe corn husks and peanut shells, "poultry protein products" to describe hydrolyzed chicken feathers, and "processed animal protein" for ground bones.

A rather unsavory business for a supposedly savory business, I would say. The Humane Society of the United States and the American Veterinary Holistic Medical Association were strongly opposed.

According to the International Journal for the Study of Animal Problems, such vagueness in labeling could cause serious health problems among sensitive pets. Furthermore, said the journal, the labeling of animal byproducts that are actually of little or no nutritional value as "protein" not only misleads the public but can also be detrimental to animal health.

All those percentages of protein, fat and carbohydrates on the container provide no useful information on biological values, that is, the actual utilization quality of ingredients. Can your animals really use the food — digest it, and process it into the necessities of life?

For much of it, no way. Animal "protein" such as feathers, hair, beaks and claws are virtually indigestible yet such ingredients contribute to the total protein percentage in the "Guaranteed Analysis" that appears on the package. An authority on cat nutrition once estimated that only about 50 percent of the protein in "good" diets is actually utilized. What about diets that are less than good?

Fats may consist of rancid oils lacking essential fatty acids and certain fiber contents may act as irritants.

The fact is that the "Guaranteed Analysis" on the label is no guarantee at all that the contents are nourishing. In the opinion of many veterinarians, the extra protein and harsh ingredients place an overload on the kidneys, liver, intestines and other organs involved in bodily food processing. Loose stools, gassy bowels, direct irritation to the intestinal tract, and a whole assortment of allergic reactions and illnesses are typical results when the organs can no longer cope.

For sure, the poor-quality excess protein over the long-run is a prescription for kidney disease. The kidneys have to process and excrete the toxins and nitrogenous waste products from protein breakdown. But nature never designed canine or feline kidneys to handle the volume of impurities that comes their way. The result is fatigued, irritated, damaged and deteriorated kidneys after several years of life. Scar tissue replaces healthy tissue and cannot perform the normal task of filtration. Waste products are retained in the body instead of being excreted. These poisons often collect in skin tissue and cause shabby coats and itchy, dry or scaly skin, a situation that mimics an allergic dermatitis. Left untreated, the toxic buildup leads to vomiting, loss of appetite, uremic poisoning and death.

Kidney disease should be a prime suspect when an animal seems constantly thirsty and drinks large amounts of water. The signs also include pale, often colorless, urine. Excretion is more frequent than usual.

In my practice I see many cats and dogs with diet-caused kidney disease too advanced to treat.

Dr. Mark Morris, Jr., one of the country's leading veterinary nutritionists, has stated that a high protein food is "not good for your dog" and if the animal has kidney problems, "an all-meat dog food can kill him." The International Journal for the Study of Animal Problems quoted Morris as saying that all of the commercially available dog foods contain so much extra protein than what is actually required that it would take an extraordinary search to find a food with insufficient quantities. Research has clearly shown high protein diets to have an adverse effect on kidneys, the journal said.

San Jose veterinarian Wendell Belfield, in his book "How To Have A Healthier Dog," reports the case of a terrier who was fed a cheap high-protein diet and died of complete kidney shutoff and uremic poisoning.

"In a healthy animal, you should see kidneys the size of nice walnuts," said Belfield. "When I opened the dog for autopsy, I found two shriveled-up kidneys, half that size, and hard with scar tissue. I kept them in formaldehyde for many years to show clients just exactly what can happen to animals fed an inferior diet."

A CHEMICAL FEAST

The manufacturing process also includes a hefty infusion of some of the foremost chemical additives of our time. There's sodium nitrite, to prevent fading of colors and make meat products look a healthy blood-red. There's

Red Dye 40 to create a fresh, meaty appearance. Not that the animal would notice the color. Cats and dogs are thought to be colorblind. The cosmetics are all for you. It's important you think the product looks good enough to eat. Er, rather, that it looks good enough to buy.

Sodium nitrite and Red dye 40 have long been linked to cancer or birth defects in laboratory animals. They are banned in some countries, but not here. Two widely used preservatives — butylated hydroxyanisole (BHA) and butylated hydroxytoluene (BHT) — have been associated with liver damage, fetal abnormalities, metabolic stress and increased cholesterol in some laboratory testing. They also have a questionable relationship to cancer.

No doubt you've heard of the "Chinese Restaurant Syndrome." That's where sensitive individuals will experience headaches, feverish flushes and rapid heartbeat after eating a Chinese meal. The cause is monosodium glutamate (MSG), a flavor enhancer used liberally in Chinese restaurants. The very same MSG is also used in a number of the most popular dog and cat foods.

So, too, is sodium metabisulfite, a preservative, which has been making headlines lately for its ability to cause brain damage, difficulty swallowing, weakness, loss of consciousness and other major grief in sensitive humans. What is it causing in sensitive animals?

A vast array of chemicals are pumped into commercial pet food to extend shelf life and make the products attractive and tasty. "Few foods are so liberally laced with artificial flavors as pet foods," reported Consumers Digest several years ago. The magazine quoted a source in the additive industry as saying that phony flavors is the only way to get pets to eat the quality-poor food.

Do you feed your pets semi-moist products? The version for dogs contains as much as 25 percent of the contents as sugar! The sweet stuff gives it taste and also prevents bacterial contamination. It may be also creating canine sugar junkies. In addition to semi-moist products, treats and snacks are often loaded with sugar, syrups and artificial sweeteners.

Cats don't have the sweet tooth that dogs do, so the semi-moist feline version contains propylene glycol as a substitute for sugar. Propylene glycol, an iffy additive known to cause puzzling irregularities in the blood of cats, belongs to a chemical family that is used in anti-freeze, oils and waxes. In dogs, it is known to cause a severe skin inflammation, hair loss and even death.

Semi-moist is a near-total chemical concoction that many veterinarians regard as pure garbage. I have seen it lead to cardiac failure in older dogs with heart problems, and cause many cases of diarrhea, vomiting and allergic reactions.

Too much salt in the human diet is a well-known problem. But did you realize that there's too much salt in semi-moist and other highly-processed pet diets as well? It's a common additive, used as a preservative to prevent spoilage of meats. When listed on the label, as much as 6 percent of the formulation may consist of salt.

Too much salt (and sugar, too) can irritate the stomach and the intestines. It can create an abnormal thirst that promotes an excess drinking of water. Animals will sometimes bloat up with so much liquid they vomit. Then they will bloat up again on water and vomit once again in a continuing cycle that drains their bodies of essential minerals. I have treated many an animal, weak and near death — hapless victims of a disastrous diet.

Industry usage of additives is inadequately controlled by government. Safety testing is generally conducted by the individual manufacturers themselves and not by independent researchers. And there are seemingly as many loopholes in safety regulations as there are additives — and there are thousands of them.

Consider this: The U.S. Government's General Accounting Office issued a report in 1979 indicating that all commercially-sold meat is contaminated to some degree with chemicals. Something like "fourteen percent of the dressed raw meat and poultry sold in supermarkets might contain illegal residues of chemicals suspected of causing cancer, birth defects or other toxic effects," the report said.

Six years later, in 1985, the Food and Drug Administration was taken to task by a Congressional committee for failing to protect consumers from exposure to dangerous drugs that are fed to animals and can turn up in meat, dairy products and eggs.

Such is the freightening situation for human quality food — food that you and I eat. Imagine the degree of contamination in pet foods.

One FDA toxicologist expressed "a great deal of concern" to veterinarian Wendell Belfield that among the questionable things going into pet foods are "the toxic agricultural chemicals — the pesticides and herbicides — killing numbers of livestock every day."

Such animals are processed for pet food, livestock and poultry feed, the toxicologist said, and nobody knows how much of the poisons are surviving the processing. While sterilization will eliminate the microbes contained in contaminated food, most agricultural chemicals will survive the high temperature involved in processing, he added.

Medical science cannot possibly keep pace with the rapid progress of profit-motivated food science. Nor can our animals. They did not evolve on the deluge of chemicals they now get during a lifetime of eating a totally man-made diet.

Unfortunately, the public and most veterinarians receive their entire nutritional information from manufacturers whose primary interest is sales.

After a study of pet foods during the 1970s, Dr. Paul M. Newberne of the Department of Nutrition and Food Science at the Massachusetts Institute of Technology, had this to say: "Much of the information...on how best to feed your pet...is misleading and primarily designed to sell a product...often with very little if any supporting evidence to back the claims made by the manufacturer. The pet-owning public and in many cases the veterinary profession has thus been at the mercy of the mass media advertising, often to the detriment of the health of the animal and increased cost to the client.''

In a highly critical 1979 article on pet food, Frances Sheridan Goulart of Consumers Digest issued this caveat: ''There is mounting evidence that a lifetime of eating commercial pet foods can shorten your pet's life, make him fatter than he ought to be and contribute to the development of such increasingly common disorders as cystitis and stones (in cats), glaucoma and heart disease (in dogs), diabetes, lead poisoning, rickets and serious vitamin-mineral deficiencies (in both cats and dogs).''

And in a 1980 book for cat owners, pet columnist Jean Burden described the difficulties encountered by the modern cat trying to adapt to man-made environment and food: ''It doesn't always wholly succeed. Sometimes its teeth fall out at an early age; sometimes it gives birth to stunted kittens. All because of poor nutrition.''

For years I have been watching the pet food market with growing concern. And what I see are antiquated and improper formulations full of chemical additives, questionable ingredients that cannot be utilized, and inadequate levels of vitamins and minerals.

Today's food is daily becoming more inadequate and unacceptable for today's animals. The criterion for purchase is no longer what food is best, but rather what food will cause less problems.

3

Food Allergies — Trouble By The Mouthful

Where's the beef? they say. I'll tell you. It's at the very top of my "Allergic HIT List" of foods that cause our pets the most problems.

Beef is fed so frequently in so many ways, shapes and forms, that it's the No. 1 allergic hitman by a big margin.

Beef is beef, you say. Steaks and prime roasts. Whatya mean different ways, shapes and forms?

It's unlikely you are feeding choice cuts to your animals. More likely you are feeding commercial formulations that include beef from condemned parts and byproducts. These are the typical forms of beef generally processed into canned, semi-moist and dry kibble products, into pet snacks such as biscuits and bone treats, into rawhide chew sticks, and into meat sauce, meat meal and bone meal.

These entities all have the beef antigen — the offending protein molecule — and it is literally flooding the digestive tracts of animals everywhere.

Is your animal diabetic? Is it on insulin? Is the insulin from a beef source? If your animal is sensitive to beef it may also be sensitive to beef insulin as well. The insulin may therefore be totally ineffective for the diabetes yet effective in an undesirable way — provoking allergic reactions.

Is your animal on thyroid therapy? Is the thyroid replacement from beef? If so, it may not be effective at all if the animal is sensitive to beef.

Are you giving your animals supplements or coat enhancers containing a beef source? Read your labels.

Out in nature animals can follow the heeding of instinct and choose their own meals and snacks. But pets are beholden, both benefactor and victim of their master's decisions. And too often they receive the same food day after day, can after can, sack after sack. And in those cans and sacks are usually meat and meat byproducts in one form or another.

Actor Bill Shatner, the Captain Kirk of Star Trek fame, and his actress wife Marcy, are long-time clients of mine and can tell you first-hand about beef allergy. It almost killed "Heidi," their pet Doberman.

About ten years ago, "Heidi" developed a sudden hind leg paralysis. The incident occurred while I was on vacation and the Shatners took the dog to see another veterinarian. "Heidi" was diagnosed as having a serious spinal condition affecting her legs. She was in obvious pain. The veterinarian thought she should be put to sleep.

The Shatners were extremely attached to "Heidi." They said they wanted to get a second opinion, so they waited a few days until I returned. The X-rays showed that the first veterinarian had made a mistake. There was no spinal problem. But there was a horrible gas problem. The dog's abdomen was severely distended with gas and she was dragging her hind legs. The pressure was apparently causing a referred-type of pain in her legs much the same way that angina (heart-related chest pain) in people can cause pain in the left arm.

I suspected "Heidi" was having a common intestinal reaction to a food allergen. I had seen many cases of gassy bloating as a result of food allergy. As in this case, sometimes the hind legs are painfully affected to the point where the animal appears paralyzed, thus imitating a sign of disc disease for which dogs are often put to sleep.

I gave "Heidi" some medication to soothe her gut and sent her home with a prescription for a non-meat diet. Within two weeks she was dramatically better and walking normally again.

Moreover, within three months, Marcy told me that "Heidi" had undergone major changes. The dog was five-years-old at the time but now frolicked with the vigor of a puppy. Her coat improved and her personality blossomed.

The Shatners maintained the dog on a non-meat diet for the rest of her life. She enjoyed radiant health almost until the end. She died at the ripe old age of 14.

So impressive were the changes "Heidi" made those ten or so years ago that we came to name the diet after her — the "Heidi Diet." I'll give you the details and recipe in Chapter Fourteen.

The Shatner case represents a typical finding about food allergy. It's this: animals often become sensitive to the foods they eat the most frequently. "Heidi" had been receiving a steady stream of beef in her diet. At the time, the Shatners felt they were feeding her the best possible diet. Unfortunately, as things turned out, they learned that the continuing volume of beef was overcoming the animal's ability to cope. One day, the dog's body finally said "no more."

It is important to note that it is usually the old diet, the food the animal has been eating perhaps for years, that most often becomes offensive and triggers allergic reactions. When I mention to clients that diet may be involved in a particular problem, they sometimes react quite defensively.

"Well, I've been feeding the same food for years without any problem," they will say. That very admission is a strong clue for me. Exposure to the same food over a prolonged period can certainly do an animal in.

Many animals can handle small or moderate amounts of a problem food.

But when you heap the chow in the doggy or kitty bowl then you are often overloading the threshold. Again, let's use beef as an example. The food becomes an allergen because of the frequency it is fed. There's beef in the main course, beef in the chewsticks, and more beef in the snack. It's too much exposure. The animal cannot handle it all. The more one-sided the diet the greater the chance for rejectivity to occur earlier on in life.

The constant bombardment of beef is why I will routinely take many sick animals off a beef diet. Often they will recover just on the basis of this one simple measure.

I recall one dog — "Archie" was his name, a three-year-old mixed breed — who suffered chronically with stomach and intestinal upset. Occasionally he would break out with severe facial swelling. We took him off beef and the intestinal problem disappeared. However, the swelling returned from time-to-time. It turned out that he was still getting an occasional shot of beef in the form of pastrami. His owner was a New Yorker who loved his deli and enjoyed sharing it with "Archie." Pastrami, of course, is yet another form of beef.

Animals can develop an intestinal problem over a period of time, or, like "Heidi," experience an acute onset where there may be a tremendous pocket of gas or vomiting or diarrhea. Burbly stomachs, gassiness and loose stools on a regular basis are tip-offs that an animal isn't handling the diet well.

Based on years of watching and treating food allergies, I created my "Allergic HIT List" of major food offenders. HIT stands for High In Trouble. These are the foods I have observed causing the most trouble. You may have a cat or a dog that is sensitive to any one or several of them.

THE ALLERGIC HIT LIST
Dogs

1. Beef and beef byproducts
2. Milk
3. Yeast, yeast-containing foods, brewer's yeast (as given to animals for supposed flea protection).
4. Corn and corn oil
5. Pork.
6. Turkey.
7. Eggs.
8.. Fish and fish oils.
9. Wheat and wheat byproducts (when in combination with 1-8.

Cats

1. Beef and beef byproducts.
2. Tuna.
3. Milk.
4. Yeast and yeast products.
5. Pork.
6. Turkey.

Let's look at these frequent offenders in greater detail. Later, in Chapter Fourteen, I will discuss the safest foods along with some hypoallergenic recipes you can either prepare yourself or purchase for your animals.

● Milk. There is a great misconception about cow's milk, thought to be "Mother Nature's perfect food." It may be perfect — but only if you are a calf.

I know of one Texas physician who studied the effects of milk for over 40 years and concluded that it is poorly absorbed, impairs the uptake of nutrients, stimulates excess mucous production, and leads to a host of problems including diarrhea, weight gain, chronic fatigue and allergic reactions.

Textbooks on human food allergies list milk as the most offending of foodstuffs. One study in New York revealed that 25 percent of infants fed cow's milk will develop one or more allergies. A recent study in England indicated that milk caused 30 percent of headaches experienced by a group of schoolchildren. For most people around the world, drinking what in this country would be considered normal amounts of milk past infancy is likely to result in sickness.

The situation with our pets is pretty much the same, despite all those images of cats contently lapping up bowls of milk. Afterward, the cat may rush behind a bush or barn and throw up.

In my experience, perhaps as many as 80 percent of our cats and dogs, no matter what age, cannot tolerate cow's milk. After drinking it they usually have gassy stomachs, vomiting, loose stool or diarrhea. It doesn't matter what form the milk is in — raw, low fat or non-fat. However, animals do seem to have a greater tolerance to cottage cheese and other cheeses.

● Yeast. Another common misconception is to supplement cats and dogs with brewer's yeast, thinking it will protect them from fleas. In my opinion, it doesn't. What it will often do, however, is cause skin allergies.

"Abba,"a two-year-old Siamese cat, was brought to my clinic with red, inflamed ears and hair loss over the tail base. I learned the owner was giving the animal brewer's yeast. I suggested she change to a hypoallergenic diet and stop the yeast.

In a week's time, she reported the condition of the skin was improving. After another couple of weeks she said hair was starting to grow back on the cat's hind end.

Within a month she and "Abba" were back in my office. It seems that a friend of her's — a "health nut" — had resold her on the virtues of brewer's yeast. The old skin problems were coming back. The owner now became a believer. She kept the cat off brewer's yeast and the condition cleared up. She was even able to resume his standard diet.

I see many animals in my practice who have difficulty with yeast. Later, in Chapter Twelve I will explain why yeast doesn't work against fleas.

● Wheat and corn. In a sensitive animal, wheat and corn products can induce vomiting and itchy, scratchy skin. Wheat, of course, is a major allergen among humans, ranking right up there with milk. Corn is also problematic, but less so.

In pet foods, these grains are used as cheap fillers and sources of carbohydrate. Often they are the single largest ingredients in the product.

Many breeders are aware of the highly allergenic effects of wheat and will feed a corn-based product instead. In formulations that contain both grains, a sensitive animal is getting a double dose of trouble.

It is interesting to note that corn is the number one ingredient in many cat food products. What's curious about this is that the cat was domesticated about three thousand years ago as a protector of grainaries precisely because it refused to eat grain. Only within the last twenty years or so has the cat been eating grain. This latter-day development has absolutely nothing to do with feline evolution or dietary preference, but rather with the discovery by food manufacturers that if you mask corn with animal fat, a cat will eat it. The cheap price and plentiful supply of corn is most likely a primary motivating force here.

● Tuna. A very appealing flavor and popular food with cats. The high exposure results in frequent skin problems and intestinal upset as well as contributing to pancreas, liver and kidney problems and urinary tract blockage.

● Pork and turkey. Come Christmas and Thanksgiving, there's a predictable flood of sick animals at veterinary clinics everywhere. It's obvious that the festive spirit has extended to the family pet, who receives his or her share of the bounty in the form of leftover turkey and ham.

Problem is that many animals can't tolerate turkey or pork. For some, a nibble is enough to make them ill with vomiting or diarrhea.

Turkey is probably too expensive for pet food manufacturers to use routinely in their formulations. Otherwise we might see more allergic reactions to it. From my experience, the incidence of turkey reactions tend to follow a holiday schedule.

As well as pure allergic reactions there have also been cases of classic holiday overeating — pets perhaps following their masters' example. I'll never forget one sick Beagle who had been particularly gluttinous. I was told he had downed all the yuletide turkey and ham tossed his way. For dessert, he had found and finished an entire box of See's chocolates.

Another Beagle once got thoroughly sick when he ate a small turkey hen, pop-up thermometer included.

Many times following holiday celebrations leftover ham bones are stored — and forgotten — in refrigerators. People will sometimes discover the ham weeks afterward and give it to Fido. As a result of eating the ham, the animal may become violently ill, with vomiting and diarrhea. What happens is that a powerful toxin forms on the meat after two weeks or so and can cause intestinal upheaval.

I have also found that high-fat foods such as pork can elicit damaging reactions in the pancreas. I remember one woman who fed her dog three strips of bacon every morning. It eventually killed the animal. Autopsy showed an inflamed, hemmorhagic pancreas.

● Eggs. Many people like to feed their animals raw eggs. It may not be such a good idea. Raw egg whites contain avidin, a protein that renders biotin, one of the B complex vitamins, unavailable to the body. A lack of biotin can result in skin problems, among other things. Cooking neutralizes the avidin. So if you are going to feed eggs, serve them cooked please. But in doing so be aware that eggs can be allergenic, in particular the whites.

One of the poodles in my practice is a dramatically egg-sensitive animal. In his case if he eats eggs his face will swell up grotesquely.

Years ago, eggs were used in preparing distemper vaccines for dogs. Eggs were dropped from the formulation, however, after they were found to be causing allergic reactions in many animals.

● Other food allergens I have seen with some frequency in my practice include peas, beans, nuts, shellfish, chocolate, fresh fruit, grapes, pineapple, tomatoes, cabbage, chard, broccoli, cauliflower, mushrooms, and spices.

Just how little it takes to cause an allergic reaction is dramatized by a case I had involving a dog with a chronic dermatitis, a skin rash. We brought the dog into the hospital and put him on a special diet and he did fine. The rash cleared up. I sent the dog home after a week and told the owners to maintain that diet and not to stray off it.

Well, the animal was back two weeks later with the same rash even though the owner swore he was following the strict diet.

What happened?

Our owner liked to munch on peanuts when he watched TV in the evenings. Innocently, he would toss a few peanuts to his pet sprawled at his feet. And that was enough. Just a few peanuts a week. The dog was so sensitive that his skin rash returned in full bloom just from this minimum exposure.

I recall a terrier who was deathly allergic to chicken. She almost died when a housekeeper, who hadn't been informed of the chicken ban, tossed the dog a slice of chicken one day.

● Another important point to keep in mind regards the chemicals that accompany food. These can intensify or wholly activate an allergic reaction. The list includes the endless array of artificial colors, artificial flavors, artificial sweeteners, preservatives, stabilizers, etc., used in the manufacturing process. It includes the drugs, hormones and anti-biotics used to fatten feed animals. And it may also include pesticides and insecticides applied to those animals and which have survived processing to reach the feeding bowl.

● Mold can also be an allergic turn on. And it doesn't just stem from food that's going bad.

"Mickey" is a Collie I treated for allergies and he seemed to be doing fine on a special diet that eliminated many of the common allergens. When his owner, an artist, moved to an old farmhouse, the dog suddenly started biting and scratching his skin and developed severe diarrhea. This happened despite maintenance on the same good diet.

We finally tracked the problem down to mold present in the rather antiquated plumbing system. The dilemma was solved with distilled water.

4

Why Are Foods Allergenic?

Classic allergies involve abnormal and symptom-producing reactions of the immune system. Intolerances involve physical reactions to environmental substances that interfere with normal bodily functions.

In dealing with food problems, everybody has a favorite term. Allergies. Intolerances. Sensitivities. Hypersensitivities.

The name is really academic. Call it whatever you like. The bottom line is still trouble whenever you or your animal eat certain foods. Not only can food cause disease by itself but it also can act as a priming agent to increase sensitivity to other allergens. Signs can occur at any time, from a few weeks of age on up to old age.

A sensitive animal is one who overreacts or experiences an abnormal reaction or illness from eating certain food. And certain foods seem to elicit a greater reaction than others. But why in one particular animal and not in another? Why is one animal's meat the next animal's poison? How is it that Cat A eats a can of tuna and is fine, yet Cat B breaks out with a skin rash? How is it Dog A eats Brand X kibble and seems to do fine, yet the dog next door gets violent diarrhea from the same food?

The answers are not simple nor are there always answers. There can be a number of possibilities involved. Let me try to make as clear as possible what is not really a fully understood chain of events.

THE INTESTINAL WAR ZONE

In my clinical experience I have found that the majority of the sensitive animals, when tested, have an imbalance in the antibody responsible for law and order in the intestinal tract. The name of this antibody is IgA, standing for immunoglobulin A. It is an antibody found throughout the mucous membrane linings of the body, including the lining of the stomach and intestines.

IgA is produced by a systemic army of protective white blood cells, lymphocytes by name. It's easier if you think of them as soldier cells because they do battle with "foreign invaders" throughout the body, such as bacteria and virus. Among the various "weapon systems" utilized by these lymphocytes are specialized antibodies. They act as roadblocks or bio-chemical bullets. IgA is one of them.

In the gut lining, these soldier cells occupy front-line positions, ever on alert for the impurities and bacteria that arrive with the food. It's their job to try and neutralize such contaminants and block passage through the intestinal wall into the bloodstream.

If all is well, a multiplicity of efficient digestive processes are going on at this time. Food is being broken down by visceral secretions into basic nutrient components for absorption.

However, a genetic biochemical defect common to many, many pets may be undermining the function of the lymphocytes. As a result, these soldier cells may react wildly, producing either too few, too many or totally impotent IgA antibodies. This erratic action can interfere with digestive processing and also irritate the intestinal lining.

Among other things, the disorder created allows many impure and toxic ingredients or improperly digested foods to enter the bloodstream. Once inside, they can act as irritating allergens — "foreign invaders" — and/or put a burden on filtering organs such as the liver and kidneys to eliminate them.

As things stand anyway, ingested food may require prolonged processing because of the impurities and unnatural combinations. This extra labor and churning further irritates the intestinal walls, creating more turmoil and more entry for impurities. You get the gas buildup. You get the burbly stomach. Loose stool. Diarrhea. Vomiting. And then from the endless mechanical and chemical churning and irritation of the lining, the blood comes.

In a manner of speaking, a war zone has been created in the gut.

SKIN — EXTERNAL SPOKESMAN FOR INTERNAL AFFAIRS

Veterinarians treat more skin disorders than any other problem, according to a national survey. Although it doesn't receive as much recognition as skin-related flea allergy, food allergy can be just as troublesome to the skin.

Intestinal turmoil permits many allergens and impurities to enter the bloodstream. Certain cells in the body — called mast cells — are sensitive to this unwelcome traffic and they react by secreting histamine, a name familiar to all of you.

The histamine has an "open sesame" effect on the walls of the tiniest blood vessels, making them more permeable. Blood now seeps into the adjacent tissue through the porous walls, causing damaging chemical reactions, irritation, inflammation, and itchiness. The animal will respond to these local disturbances by scratching, chewing and biting — making the situation even worse.

The mast cells are located in greatest number just below the skin in and around the ears, around the eyes, on the chest and abdomen, above the tail base and on the feet. Here, on the skin, are the major surface impact areas where allergic reactions — so-called allergic dermatitises — are most frequently seen. Frenzied licking of paws or scratching of any of these areas are pretty sure signs of a food allergy.

"Billy" was an orange tabby cat who developed occasional thickened and inflamed ears. He would scratch so hard at them that he created what on humans would be called cauliflower ears. Blood and serum would enter the space between the skin and the cartilage of the ear, creating an extremely unsightly looking animal.

In this case, "Billy" was highly sensitive to tuna. The owner had a stepson who was very fond of the cat and whenever he came to visit he would bring some fresh tuna. It was after the visits that the scratching would start. After two of three incidents, we were able to pinpoint the problem to tuna.

Lick granuloma is a frequent skin affliction usually occurring on the legs and feet of dogs. Veterinarians usually attribute it to boredom: the dog is pent up and has nothing to do but lick, bite and chew what is obviously a nagging itchiness. The constant mouthing creates inflammation and large thickened strawberry-sized wounds.

I see this problem often as a form of food allergy which has stimulated the large cluster of mast cells in the legs and feet.

"Buck" was a black labrador who had suffered from these lick granulomas on all four legs and paws. Standard treatment hadn't worked. He had been injected with cortisone directly under the granulomas, been given oral cortisone, and various ointments. His legs had been bandaged for five weeks and one of those Elizabethan restraining collars put around his neck.

When the bandages came off the legs were much improved. However, "Buck" immediately began the frenzied licking and chewing again and soon turned his legs into a bloody mess.

The animal was referred to me. I found out he was eating a high potency kibble product containing seven of the most common allergic foods for dogs. I recommended he be taken off the kibble and started on a hypoallergenic diet. No other therapy was used.

Within five days the licking, chewing and biting stopped. Within three weeks, the wounds healed. And two weeks later we saw hair growing back on the sites. The improvement was dramatic.

Dachshunds, English Bulldogs and Huskies are known to be susceptible to interdigital cysts, bubble-like growths that form between the toes. Boxers get them sometimes, too. I've seen dozens of poor dogs chronically crippled with this painful condition, their paws swollen to twice normal size.

When these cysts are opened and drained they are sterile inside. There is no infection. There has been no foreign body puncture. So how do you treat it? Again, I regard this as a mast cell-histamine release problem triggered by food allergy and I have had many, many animals totally liberated from these cysts simply by placing them on hypoallergenic diets.

UNHOLY, UNNATURAL MIXTURES

The reasons why certain foods act as allergens are in many cases speculative. Surely, one can put forward the argument that our pets did not evolve on the unnatural configurations of commercial food.

Look at the labels of some of the products out there. Can they possibly have any relationship with the food that cats and dogs ate over centuries and millenia? The bodies and brains of these animals have been genetically programmed to utilize certain foods. I doubt if this programming includes the man-made mush they are fed today.

Most commercial combinations are pure science fiction. An animal perhaps may be able to tolerate beef and corn by themselves, but when you combine the two such as in a kibble, then tolerance takes a tumble.

Ingredients are often grossly impure, their taste and appearance "enhanced" by a conglomeration of chemicals for which there is absolutely no evidence for long-term safety.

I frankly feel that much of the commercial pet food on the market is so alien, so multiply altered, so chemically-laden, that only the strongest of animals can remain healthy on it over a lifetime.

Too much of any one food — such as beef — can overload the fragile system in a sensitive animal's gut. Some creature may tolerate perhaps only 2-3 grams (there are about 450 in a pound) of an offending food without reacting, but give him 4 grams and you overwhelm the threshold, causing signs of overt disease. Infinitesimal amounts can indeed light the fuse.

There can also be a seasonal connection here. An animal may tolerate an allergenic food during the winter, but when the insects and pollens of spring and summer enter the picture, tolerance may vanish. A summation effect, that is, the combination of food and environmental allergens, can throw an animal into allergic episodes.

If you determine a seasonal pattern you may do your animal a great favor by feeding him a low protein, additive-free, hypoallergenic diet. That can free the weapons of the immune system to pour all their firepower on the insects and pollens at hand.

Dr. Marshall Mandell, of Norwich, Connecticut, is one of this country's outstanding clinical investigators into environmental medicine and allergies. In his book, "Dr. Mandell's 5-Day Allergy Relief System," he describes the chemical situation as it applies to humans.

Mandell asks the question why should a person be allergic to anything that he eats, drinks or inhales if all things are derived in some form from something that is part of our planet.

"The answers, we have discovered, involve mankind's increasing inability to cope with natural as well as unnatural substances in his environment,'' says Mandell.

"For hundreds of thousands of years during the course of human evolution, changes occurred much more slowly in man's natural environment than they do in the rapidly changing chemicalized and polluted world of today...

"When organic chemistry began in the nineteenth century, a whole series of combinations of chemicals were created that were never found naturally in the environment. Pesticides, herbicides, insecticides, waxes, preservatives, colorings, and additives, although they did the jobs they were designed for, (they) contaminated the environment and filled man's body with residues that were totally alien to the human system...''

Added to this growing chemical heap, continues Mandell, was proliferating contamination from automotive fuels, jet fuels, and oil and coal burning industry.

"In short, everything man eats, drinks, or inhales is now polluted with chemical agents that are foreign to his chemistry, and he is suffering the consequences of possessing a body that is incapable of handling the byproducts of his amazing chemical technology.''

According to a recent issue of the Journal of the American Medical Association, the proliferation of drugs and chemicals used in food, agriculture, and industry is so widespread it is contributing to an alarmingly increasing number of people "who are allergic to everything.''

And according to a 1981 Ford Foundation Report on nutrition in this country, there is a growing epidemic of chronic disease among Americans attributable in large part to the depleted, chemicalized and highly processed nature of our food.

The parallels — and implications — to our animal population are clear. It's even frightening when you consider that much of the food our animals are eating has been declared unfit for human consumption.

KIBBLE — A SACKFUL OF TROUBLE

More convenient. Less money. That's the positive side of kibble. After that it's all negative.

I have found that many of the animals I have treated over the years are intolerant to kibble. I believe the reason is because kibble is a concentrated collection of many of the foods that are the most allergenic for animals. Practically everything on my Allergic HIT List is found in those sacks: beef, milk, wheat, corn, yeast, fish meal, plus a bountiful array of chemical additives. There's probably some mold, hair and other impurities in there as well.

Kibble is the easiest form of food for the manufacturers to blend and hide inferior protein.

First they pressure cook all those delectable parts I mentioned in Chapter Two. Then they flavor it all, color it, dehydrate it and often blow air into it to create bigger surface particles so it looks as if you are getting bigger chunks for your money. All this means multiple adulteration to protein probably poor to start with.

The number of preservatives listed on the package is a good indicator of the quality of the protein and nutrients inside. The more preservatives, the poorer the quality. It takes more of man's ingenuity to maintain the shelf life. The greater the decomposition of a corpse, the more embalming fluid you need to make it look pretty.

The dehydration of this product eliminates moisture and that can increase the impact of an allergen. Water acts as a diluter of allergens. If little moisture is present the allergen is likely to be in a more potent, concentrated form. Thus, the allergens found in kibble are generally more numerous and more concentrated than in canned or semi-moist food.

Most pet food manufacturers employ sales gimmicks to enhance sales. Over the years one of the most effective gimmicks has been the promotion of so-called high protein kibble. The makers splash high protein all over the packaging. You, the consumer, think you are getting some real high powered chow for your animal. And you go for it. Every time. You buy the lie. What you are getting is a clever cover-up that leads to a host of health problems.

A manufacturer will use an excessive amount of cheap, inferior-quality protein in order to obtain a minimum that animals can utilize. In California, for instance, the state's Food and Drug Administration requires producers to include 18 percent protein in dog kibble, knowing that animals may be able to use only 5-9 percent of it.

Cats require more protein than dogs — twice as much. According to the National Research Council, felines should receive 30 percent of their diet in the form of protein. But if only a half — in the best of products — of protein in a commercial diet is absorbed and utilized, what about the rest? What about the junk? What kind of problems is it causing?

Kibble has long been thought to be one of the causes of feline urologic syndrome (FUS). If fish or fish meal are listed on the label, this means that fish bones are included in the product. But bones contain much phosphorus and magnesium. Both can collect as gravel in the particularly narrow urinary tracts of male cats and create blockages. Excess amounts of dietary phosphorus and magnesium are undesirable. To be safe, purchase products that contain low percentages of those minerals. Ask your veterinarian for a recommendation.

Does your dog or cat burp a lot? Expel gas? Have a rumbling tummy? Loose stool? Those are signs of an irritated intestine. The food is entering the gut and the organs of digestion are finding it too coarse, too unnatural, too incompatible. High-protein kibble is often the reason for this.

Do you have an aggressive, frightened or hyperactive animal? I have often traced the problem directly to kibble. I've seen Dobies and Shepherds who you couldn't get near. The day after you change the diet they are like pussycats, wagging their tails.

SEMI MOIST — MORE TROUBLE

Semi-moist is is a horror story — the ultimate food fiction. Just read the label.

Sure, it looks great. Nice and red and moist and pliable like real hamburger meat. That's what the manufacturers want you to think it is.

But it's nothing more than the standard discards and fillers. They are tinted, flavored and processed with a genuine Hollywood flair for special effects. They use artificial colors and flavors, emulsifiers, preservatives, salt, sugar, and whatever else most humans avoid who are interested in good health.

In my opinion, semi-moist should be placed in a time capsule to serve as a record of modern food technology gone mad. When you serve it to your animal you can never be sure if it will fill up or foul up his tummy.

Years ago veterinarians on the East Coast used to recommend semi-moist as a dietary regimen to alleviate food allergies. It seems that animals with typical skin problems related to allergy would improve when fed semi-moist. But improvement was only temporary, the Easterners learned. Before long the problems would come roaring back, often with new problems added.

How could animals improve even if just temporarily when this product contains many food allergens along with a heavy-handed array of chemical additives?

I think it's because the processing of this particular product is so extreme, the ingredients so thoroughly altered, that their physical characteristics are changed. They are no longer simple beef, milk, wheat, corn or yeast proteins that the body would recognize as allergenic and possibly react to. These troublesome ingredients are now masked men, traveling the gut incognito. The body's immune system doesn't recognize them as "foreign matter." So no reactions occur.

...At least for a while.

You just can't fool the immune system too long. Eventually, the white blood cells (lymphocytes) recognize the charade and become sensitized to these ingredients. And you can then often have a whole range of reactions from vomiting and diarrhea to dry, itchy, flaky and reddened skin. Along with that is the excess drinking and urination — the tell-tale signs of the semi-moist eater. So if you switch to semi-moist and your animal seems to do well, it's probably just a honeymoon.

I frequently find semi-moist food as the cause of common allergic or allergic-like reactions. My advise is not to feed it to your animal.

CANNED FOOD

Canned food, just like like the rest of commercial pet food, may be allergenic to your animals. That's because it contains many of the food items that pets are most sensitive to.

Some animals react, usually in the form of diarrhea or vomiting, to the preservatives used in these products.

On the whole, however, animals may be somewhat less reactive to canned food. The reason being that the contents are 72-78 percent water. Thus, less than 30 percent of the contents may have allergic properties and those will be diluted by the high water volume.

WHAT'S LEFT?

Kibble. Semi-moist. Canned. What's left? you're thinking. He's torpedoed the whole marketplace.

Not quite. There are still many good products readily available through regular retail outlets and through your veterinarian.

And there are also some good simple hypoallergenic recipes for those of you who want to give your animals some home cooking.

In Chapter Fourteen I will advise you how to feed your animals the best-possible diet — one that eliminates, rather than causes, problems — and how to recognize signs of allergy to a specific food.

There is much you can do — and with little effort — to put health back into the diets of your dogs and cats.

5

Food Allergies Can Strike Anywhere

Food allergy is a missile with a multiple warhead. It can strike anywhere on the physical map — any surface, part or system. Wherever there is a weak spot. The impact area can be genetically predetermined or follow predictable patterns such as the mast cell-histamine route. And any food or chemical or combination thereof can do the trick, causing one or more reactions at any given time.

Gut and skin reactions may be the most typical but other acute, chronic or subtle diseases are also produced by food. It is a common misconception to think that food allergy affects only the intestines or skin.

Here are some of the many disorders I have traced to food. It may surprise you to think of them as food-related problems. In the beginning it surprised me as well.

BEHAVIOR

Allergens entering the system frequently affect the brain and nervous system, resulting in severe personality changes. Animals will suddenly become aggressive toward owners. Or they will become extremely timid and frightened and hide under beds or in closets or shy away when you approach them.

A typical case involved a six-month-old German Shepherd female who began snapping at the children in the house. Previously she had romped and played happily with them. Upon examination, the dog snapped at me also. I questioned the owner and learned that the animal had recently been taken off a puppy-type kibble and placed on a high protein formulation. The problem seemed related to the change in diet. I kept the dog overnight in the clinic and fed her a low protein diet. The next day the dog was a sweetheart. From then on the owner fed her a hypoallergenic diet without further incident.

Similarly, a sweet and personable three-year-old Siamese male suddenly changed into a feline Jekyll. One day, without any warning or apparent cause, he charged at the owner who was sitting in a chair at the time and bit and clawed at her leg. The cat was being fed a chicken-tuna combination along with a popular brand of kibble.

Examination revealed a high eosinophil count. Eosinophils are a type of white blood cell that race onto the scene like cavalry whenever histamine is released. I like to refer to them as "histamine busters" because they act to neutralize histamine. I have found elevated eosinophils a common accompaniment to food-mediated disorders.

We put the cat on a diet of lamb, the least offending of meats for most pets, and soon he became Mr. Nice Guy again. At a later date, the owner ran out of lamb and fed some leftover kibble to the cat. Within hours, the animal started acting strange again.

There has been precious little research by veterinarians into the dietary link to abnormal behavior. However, the human experience gives us considerable insight.

The work of the late Dr. Benjamin Feingold is familiar to many people. Feingold, an allergist, found that some children develop adverse behavioral reactions when they eat food containing chemical additives and dyes. Since his work was first published in 1973 there have been numerous subsequent investigations. Some support his findings while others are inconclusive.

In a 1978 experiment with rat pups, researchers found that a mixture of common commercial food colorings contributed to hyperactivity and impaired the performance of the animals during intelligence tests.

Dr. Richard Pitcairn, the pet columnist of Prevention Magazine, has written that hyperactive children "have often been helped by cutting out all foods with various synthetic additives, as well as many processed foods and foods which may aggravate allergies. I feel such products may well contribute to animal hyperactivity also."

EPILEPSY

Did you know that epilepsy is more common in dogs than in humans? Convulsive seizures also affect dogs far more than any other domesticated animal. But despite much investigation into possible causes, the disorder basically remains a mystery to veterinary scientists. Different researchers have linked the problem to genetics, emotional reaction, food allergies, and hormonal and biochemical influences.

Seizures range in severity from the so-called petit mal, or minimal attack, to the most serious, the grand mal. In the lesser type, an animal usually appears frightened or anxious to escape his environment. This is followed by stiffening, immobility and a rapid champing with the mouth, as if trying to remove a morsel of food with the tongue. There is often a foaming saliva. In the grand mal, there are violent spasms. The champing extends into jaw and neck muscle spasms with violent shaking of the head. The major muscles of the body become rigid. The attack subsides with a relaxation of the jaw, a running motion of the legs and often with urination and/or defecation. Afterward, for several minutes, animals have a dazed appearance.

In my opinion, food allergies should always be suspected. In my practice I always recommend that an epileptic animal be placed on a low protein hypo-allergenic diet.

Dr. Jim Wilson, a veterinarian who practices in Concord, California, had a classic case involving a three-year-old female Golden Retriever. The dog had uncontrollable epilepsy despite a maximum dosage of Primadone, a powerful anti-convulsant drug. We talked by phone about the case and I suggested feeding her a non-meat kibble. The new diet was started and no new seizures occurred. This encouraged Wilson to start weaning the dog slowly off the medication.

To this day, more than three years later, there have been no more seizures. The dog is maintained on a hypoallergenic diet and takes no medication at all. Here was an animal unable to be controlled by any drug and who was certain to be put to sleep. By treating the cause, instead of the end result, the suffering was stopped and the dog's life saved.

After I graduated veterinary school I started in private practice in Hollywood. One of my early patients there was a big white fluffy cat appropriately named "Oscar." She belonged to a struggling actress. The cat suffered from grand mal seizures and had been kept sedated for years on phenobarbital.

The owner was feeding him a standard diet of canned and dry food. I suggested she try cooking up a rice and chicken combination for the cat and see if that might help. The seizures quickly stopped and we were able to reduce the phenobarbital and then cut it out altogether. The cat did fine afterward. Something in the commercial diet was causing the epilepsy.

CHRONIC BRONCHITIS

The vast majority of bronchial cases have viral, bacterial or inhalant origins and few people would ever connect them to food. But food can indeed be the problem.

These more unusual cases may involve IgA, the antibodies located throughout the body in mucous membrane. They are in the gut, as we have just seen, and they are also in the lining of the lungs.

If there is an adrenal hormone imbalance — an irregularity I find frequently — then problems with IgA activity can occur anywhere in the body where the antibody is present. When the blood carries some of the bizarre food components through the lung tissue the IgA present may pounce on such "foreign matter" and overreact to the degree that local irritation is created. This can then lead to inflammation, rapid respiration and coughing.

"Max," a whippet, suffered terrible pneumonia-like bouts until we discovered that his problem was beef. Take him off beef and he was fine. Once, a house guest fed "Max" a hot dog, triggering a violent coughing attack that almost killed the animal.

A veterinary radiologist who used to work nearby once took X-rays of a cat who had a chronic coughing condition along with light, shallow respiration. The pictures showed lung inflammation. The case was referred to me. We attempted standard treatment with anti-biotics but to no avail. At that point I decided to look at the possibility of food involvement. I found out the cat had been eating a diet largely of tuna and beef. I recommended a switch to lamb and chicken. The cat began to make a steady improvement. Subsequent pictures showed the inflammation was gone.

CHRONIC HEPATIC (LIVER) DISEASE

Do your animals have chronic liver disease? Have they been in and out of treatment with the typical signs of listlessness, nausea, tense or distended abdomens, with jaundice in the most severe cases? Has your veterinarian said there isn't anything that can be done about it and your animal would just have to live with it?

Living with this problem is not a pleasant prospect — for you or the animal. Chronic liver disease, if unchecked, can develop into a multisystemic disorder resulting in death.

Here again is a fairly common condition I often trace to food. Food, including additives and impurities, can act allergenically as an irritant to the filtering units in the liver. Prolonged harassment of liver tissue can impair and block the gland's critical functions of processing and filtering the bloodborne foodstuffs carried from the intestines.

A standard blood test helps determine liver disease. Specifically checked are levels of liver enzymes (SGPT and SGOT) and eosinophils. High enzyme counts represent a damaged, inflamed liver — the enzymes are being dumped into the bloodstream.

A high eosinophil count is a sign of a food allergy. In dogs, a 2-8 percent eosinophil count is regarded as normal. In my experience anything over 3 percent is suggestive of a damaging allergic reaction. Cat norms are considered to be 2-12 percent but I regard anything over 5 as suspicious. When enzyme and eosinophil counts are both elevated I will treat the animal for food allergy and put it on a hypoallergenic diet.

I believe the dietary approach is an effective and conservative first step. Switch the diet for a week's time and then recheck the blood. If the counts have dropped you know you are dealing with a food-related problem. I feel this is a much safer approach than resorting immediately to a liver biopsy. The biopsy is performed in order to examine structural damage to the liver. Surgical removal of liver tissue can be a dangerous procedure. Some animals die from it.

If a persistent liver condition exists, I suggest switching to a hypoallergenic diet. This may alleviate the inflammation and clogging within the liver.

Animals often improve with this simple step. The best bet, if possible, is to cook fresh foods for the animal — such as rice, lamb and vegetables — and make sure there are no chemical additives present.

Many of the chronic liver conditions I see respond to this form of therapy. I get dramatic cures. In my mind, therefore, many cases are largely created by impure food and food allergens.

"Salty" was a large black and white cat with a huge appetite. He ate what his owner fed him, which was basically a dry kibble, and also what was available at the neighbor's, who also had cats.

Over a two-year period, "Salty" developed a half-dozen or so episodes of general malaise and vomiting, according to his owner. When she brought the cat in for diagnosis I found high liver enzyme counts and elevated eosinophils. So I suspected food was involved.

I instructed the owner to feed "Salty" a diet of baked chicken and keep him in the house for a week. This she did. When she brought the cat back he had improved greatly. Both his enzyme and eosinophil counts had returned to normal.

All was well until the woman left town for a few days. "Salty" was left to the care of a housesitter. The cat managed to slip out somehow and get into the food bowl of the cats next door. When the owner returned, "Salty" was sick again.

Back in the hospital, I tested the cat and found the same signs and same elevated counts. We put "Salty" on a restricted diet and within a week's time he was back to health.

Another vivid case I recall involved a blond Cocker Spaniel named "Felix" who had a history of skin problems. I managed to clear up his skin by putting him on a commercial lamb product. However, the animal appeared listless. I checked his blood and found the elevated liver enzymes. There was probably something in the canned lamb that was disturbing his liver. When I checked the can, sure enough, it contained BHA, a preservative. I told the woman she would have to cook for her animal because of his liver sensitivity. She prepared lamb and rice for him and he did fine afterwards.

CHRONIC PANCREATITIS

Pancreatic disease is usually regarded as one of the signs of aging. But I see it frequently in younger animals, too. I believe that dietary impurities and chemicals, and not just age, can also harm the pancreas.

The pancreas has two major functions. One is to send salvoes of digestive juices into the small intestine for breakdown of foodstuffs. The other is the secretion of insulin to help maintain a proper level of blood sugar, the body's energy fuel.

With a chronic pancreatitis, tiny ducts within the gland become irritated and inflamed. These minute canals make up a feeder system that carry pancreatic secretions along their way to the intestines. I believe local problems here are in part caused by impurities that have been absorbed into the blood-stream and, as they pass through the blood vessels in the pancreas, exert a corrosive and damaging effect.

In this disorderly situation, the digestive juices begin to back up and, destroy the host tissue. This backup impairs the specialized functions of the pancreas. At the other end of the ducts, with less digestive enzymes available, food is improperly broken down. As a result, an animal can develop nutritional deficiencies and start to lose weight despite eating normally.

You don't want the condition to become acute because when it does it can cause a painful death.

"Spanky" was a six-year-old Siamese male with a history of sporadic vomiting. When he was sick he would bring up undigested food. Then he would be listless for a day or two afterward and wouldn't eat.

During a six-month period, "Spanky" had lost a lot of weight. Lab tests revealed the presence of elevated digestive enzymes in the blood, indicative of the kind of enzyme blockage and damage I just described.

"Spanky" was horribly allergic to tuna and wasn't absorbing much of the food he could tolerate because of the shortage of digestive enzymes.

On a tuna-free diet, the cat slowly regained health and weight and eventually made a full recovery.

Dog breeds that seem to be more susceptible to pancreas problems are Miniature Schnauzers and Poodles.

KIDNEY AND BLADDER DISEASES

In Chapter Two I mentioned how food impurities and excess protein place a heavy burden on the kidneys and eventually can cause scar tissue and serious loss of function.

Food can also harm the kidneys in an animal with a malfunctioning immune system where the IgA network is awry.

In cats, particularly males, the bladder and urethra are a major source of problems. "Feline Enemy No.1," said Dr. Carl A. Osborne, of the University of Minnesota, describing the condition known as FUS — feline urologic syndrome. In a 1979 survey of veterinary hospitals, some 5 to 10 percent of cat admissions were FUS cases.

FUS involves inflammation, formation of bladder stones, and potentially fatal blockages of the narrow urethra. Unless the obstruction is removed, the poisonous wastes normally excreted in the urine can back up into the body and cause uremic poisoning.

There is no consensus among veterinary researchers on the cause of FUS. Many experts blame the high dietary levels of magnesium and phosphorus contained in some dry cat foods. The composition of the urinary tract stones and plugs is primarily mineral.

Other sources say the problem may have viral causes.

Osborne, a leading authority, writing in a 1981 veterinary journal, questioned the commonly-held idea that FUS is initiated by any single mechanism. A variety of causes may be involved, he suggested.

One of them, entirely overlooked, is the IgA factor. It's my opinion that a war zone is created in the urinary tract similar to the turbulence in the intestinal tract. The white blood cells in the mucous membranes of the urinary system are not protecting the territory. They are producing too much or too little or defective IgA, the antibody that should be protecting the mucous membranes. As the traffic of wastes spills through the system you have a chemical irritation of the lining. A fertile bed for bacteria and virus growth is created. They join up with mucous lining debris, minerals and other particulate matter to crystallize and form the stones and cystitises that cause cats so much suffering.

In Chapter Eleven I will go into greater detail on this FUS-IgA connection. Clinical studies I have done point to a significant genetic tie-in between IgA irregularity and the incidence of FUS.

I had a case once with a three-year-old Abyssinian male named "Doodles" who occasionally developed urinary tract infections and plugs. He would strain and yowl attempting to urinate and there would be blood in the urine. These are typical FUS signs.

The owner was feeding the cat a diet of chicken and tuna. From time to time she would serve "Doodles" a treat of beef heart, fresh from the butcher. She eventually realized that the incidence of urinary problems coincided with the treats. A blood test showed the cat had almost no IgA antibodies. Again, here was a case of immune imbalance compounded by a food allergy.

In dogs, Miniature Schnauzers are known to have frequent intestinal problems. They suffer from an inability to digest or tolerate certain foods. They also have more kidney and bladder infections than normal.

What is not generally appreciated here is the link between the gut and the urinary tract. From my observations we are dealing with food-related disease. On one hand you have food allergies and on the other you have a problem with IgA antibody, in the gut and in the urinary system. In examining many Miniature Schnauzers over the years I have often found this extended problem.

"Twiggy," a cute 18-month-old Schnauzer, experienced vomiting and diarrhea when her diet included many of the major food offenders, particularly beef and beef byproducts. There was also blood in the urine. On chicken and lamb she did just fine.

Once her owner had a barbecue and somebody apparently slipped "Twiggy" a hamburger. She nearly died from it. There was so much inflammation in the kidneys that an acute shutdown took place, resulting in a serious dose of uremic poisoning. Luckily, we were able to get her in time and we stabilized her after three days of treatment.

6

Missing Minerals

Mention nutrition to most people and they automatically think of vitamins. They ignore minerals.

And minerals really deserve better. After all, there are ninety-six times more minerals by weight in a body than vitamins. There could be no life without them and any bodily cell lacking in a single mineral cannot function properly.

Minerals are involved in nearly every physiological reaction. They team up with vitamins to form enzymes. They help transport oxygen in the bloodstream. They are the building materials of strong bones, tissue, teeth, nails, and hair coat.

Minerals are present in the soil, in water, even in the air. In minute amounts they are absorbed from the soil by plants. Herbivorous animals eat the plants and drink the water and in this way obtain the bulk of their mineral nutrients. Carnivores get their quota through the mineral content of the flesh they eat, the water they drink, and the sporadic greens they chew.

Much more is known about vitamin requirements than about minerals. This is true for both humans and animals. That's because nutritional science has only recently developed the technology with which to study minerals.

Veterinary science has determined that certain minerals are required for animals. For cats — calcium, phosphorus, sodium, potassium, magnesium, iron, copper, and iodine. Chlorine, manganese, zinc, sulfur, cobalt, selenium, molybdenum, flourine, chromium, silicon, and perhaps tin, nickel and vanadium are assumed to be essential. For dogs — calcium, phosphorus, iron, copper, potassium, magnesium, sodium, chlorine, iodine, manganese, zinc, selenium, and perhaps molybdenum, flourine, tin, silicon, cobalt, nickel, vanadium and chromium.

According to the National Research Council of the National Academy of Sciences, which investigates and recommends levels of nutritional intake, many minerals have not been sufficiently studied to permit establishment of precise daily requirements. Guidelines for formulating mineral intake for cats and dogs are therefore partially based on estimates and information borrowed from other species.

The National Research Council is comprised of subcommittees of experts who are responsible for periodic reviewing and updating data on the nutritional requirements for all animal species, including humans. Their findings are expressed in the so-called RDAs, or recommended daily allowances of vitamins, minerals, carbohydrates, fats and proteins.

"COMPLETE AND BALANCED"

Such recommendations are essentially minimum standards for the maintenance of adequate health. If a product claims itself to be "complete and balanced," that means the suggested serving for an animal must meet all those daily minimum requirements. And if a product makes no mention of "complete and balanced," that means the contents probably do not meet the minimum requirements.

It is important to keep the word minimum in sight at all times. The RDA suggestions and "complete and balanced" claims are nothing more than minimums. They are not optimal in any sense. We haven't evolved that far as food mavens to divine the best possible diet for ourselves, let alone our animals.

Veterinary nutritional science surely has a long way to go. Writing in a veterinary publication during the 1970s, Paul M. Newberne of MIT said that much more is known about "the minimal requirements essential to the maintenance of the dog than...about maximum or optimal requirements...The minimum requirements are just that, and cannot be construed as optimum." Moreover, he added, the requirements for special needs, such as those associated with pregnancy, growth, or illness, have not been precisely determined.

Much less is known about cat needs. That's because cats have been taken seriously by the veterinary profession only in recent years. The first comprehensive textbook on feline medicine was not published until 1964. In the past, standard treatment for dogs were often applied to cats, sometimes with no effect.

By 1981, cats were "in." That's the year Time Magazine did a cover story on feline popularity. And today there are even veterinary practices dedicated exclusively to cats. But there is still a lot we don't know about cats.

The National Research Council, in its latest review on cats, admits "that the available data are inadequate to set minimum nutrient requirements." Recommendations are "presumed" to be adequate to support maintenance and growth of the cat and "probable, but not certain," that they will also support reproduction.

Against this background, the loud and boastful nutritional claims made by pet food manufacturers always ring hollow to me. What's the fuss? The fuss, of course, is about selling merchandise. But beneath the hype, you — the consumer — should know the claims are based on little else than minimums. And these minimums of nutrient content, along with poor quality ingredients, create minimally healthy animals.

In order to meet the standards for vitamin and mineral requirements in "complete and balanced" products, manufacturers add nutrient mixtures during processing. There can be considerable nutrient loss, however, particularly of the vitamins, as a result of their sensitivity to heat, moisture, light and oxidation. Such degradation occurs during processing, and storage in warehouses, stores, and the consumer's house. Because of this reality, consciencious manufacturers will fortify their products with extra vitamins.

But overages or not, a sack of dry food, for instance, is going to be considerably less fresh and nutritious after it has been opened fifteen or twenty times than when you first bought it from the store. A large sack of kibble may be the most economical. However, the longer storage and repeated opening results in dwindling nutrition.

The most sensitive vitamins are the B complex group. Veterinarian researchers and practitioners have traced serious problems directly to insufficient B vitamins in the diet. Hyperactivity and aggressiveness in dogs and cats can sometimes be remedied by B complex supplementation.

VITAMIN THERAPY DISAPPOINTING

Over the years I have had just so-so results with vitamin therapy. Allergies have not responded very well at all. In fact, supplementation with B complex vitamins can frequently make allergies worse. The reason: yeast is the most common commercial source of natural B complex vitamins and yeast is a leading allergen. If you supplement B complex, you are probably better off with a synthetic form.

I have my doubts about many of the vitamin products that are available on the market, particularly the most inexpensive brands. I feel that price and quality are directly related. If you buy a cheap vitamin you are likely getting a product that is wholly or partly inactive. Some products are not only inactive but may also be rancid. For these reasons I usually steer away from purely vitamin supplements.

I do believe in vitamin C. It can indeed be helpful in many ways for many animals. Among other things, vitamin C contributes directly to adrenal health and function. However, I have found that it has a reduced impact if an animal has genetically-damaged adrenal glands. This is a widespread defect I will be talking about in upcoming chapters.

My experience with mineral supplementation has been consistently good. I have been able to help something like ten percent of all the allergy cases I see with this simple therapy alone.

This positive effect doesn't surprise me. I strongly suspect that commercial pet food contains inadequate mineral levels.

The 1981 Ford Foundation report on nutrition in America explains how modern farming methods alone account for much lost nutritional content of food:

"Through intensive farming, poor crop management, erosion and other abusive factors, the soil in which our crops are raised has been seriously depleted of nutrients.

"The increasing use of pesticides has left harmful residues on crops and has further destroyed the soil by killing earthworms and other necessary organisms.

"Most produce is harvested before ripening to protect it during shipping; yet the ripening process on the plant is essential to high nutrient density in food."

Such practices rob the food chain of naturally-occurring essential vitamins and minerals. Thus the food you and your animal eat is shortchanged. Illness, from subtle to severe, can result.

With livestock and feed animals, the intake of minerals depends wholly on the geography. In certain areas there are known deficiencies. Supplementation is a must in order to prevent disease.

Over the years veterinarians have traced deficiency diseases to a wide number of minerals. They include nitrogen, phosphorus, calcium, potassium, magnesium, sodium, iron, chlorine, copper , manganese, zinc, molybdenum, cobalt, iodine and selenium.

Mineral research is a dynamic, rapidly developing science. Sophisticated techniques are being honed to probe the biological role of so-called trace minerals, the micro-nutrients present in infinitesimal amounts in the environment. These include dozens of lesser known minerals with such exotic names as yttrium, niobium, ruthenium, tellurium, scandium, osmium, dysprosium, gadollinium and praseodymium.

Any one of these unheralded substances could be a vital missing link in deficient soil, and the difference between health or disease, even at one part per million or less, which is how many of these minerals are present in food.

The body's immune system is a particularly complex network that relies on optimal nutrition for good function. If all the ingredients are not present, the system will not work as it should. A shortage of minerals can also effect the body's enzyme system that is responsible for countless numbers of biochemical reactions. Allergy or allergy-like conditions can occur when either of these systems fail to receive proper nutrition.

MINERALS TO THE RESCUE

I have found mineral deficiencies may be involved in many common disorders suffered by cats and dogs. I didn't reach this conclusion through sophisticated analysis but through the simple medium of supplementing the diets of animals with a trace mineral formula containing some seventy-two of these micro-nutrients.

Based on observations involving some three thousand seven hundred dogs and nine hundred cats, I found that trace mineral supplementation over a six-month period can help in these ways:

● Darker, thicker hair coat with increased lustre.

● Reduced scratching.

● Reduced flakiness of skin.

● Better maintenance of body weight with reduced caloric intake.

● In geriatric cats and dogs, increased activity, weight gain, and improved condition of hair coat.

● Animals with heavy flea and fly infestations appeared to be less attractive to insects after three weeks of supplementation.

● Improvement in general health.

Supplementation with a multiple nutrient of this sort is clearly a shotgun approach. Attempting to determine individual deficiencies is not within the realm of a clinician; it is the reserve of the academic researcher. Nevertheless, the trace mineral approach has often been effective alone or in conjunction with other dietary modifications. I have found it also enhances standard therapy in treating many conditions.

In dogs I have found it helpful in controlling food allergies, flea allergy dermatitis, exocrine pancreatic deficiency, endocrine-immune imbalances, chronic active hepatitis and inhalant allergies. In cats it has helped for milliary dermatitis, food allergy, flea allergy dermatitis, chronic active hepatitis, leukemia and infectious peritonitis.

I have had quite a few cases where vitamin supplements, special diets and standard medication weren't working satisfactorily until I added the trace minerals.

Just as a footnote I might mention that studies done elsewhere with the particular trace mineral formula I use in my practice has shown it to increase the muscle mass of laboratory animals and increase the mineralization — and therefore strength — of the bones. Supplemented to the diets of Idaho trout, it has increased overall weight by up to 20 percent.

Later, in Chapter Fifteen, I will discuss the formula further and tell you how to use it.

THE ZINC PROBLEM

Zinc is an essential mineral under intense scientific study these days. It is vital to the healing process, the production of enzymes, the maintenance of healthy hair coat and skin, and a well-functioning immune system and resistance to and disease.

A serious zinc problem exists in this country today. In part it is related to farming methods — the soil in over thirty states has been declared zinc-deficient by the U.S. Department of Agriculture. The primary reason is overuse of chemical fertilizers.

In recent years, veterinarians have identified a number of allergy-like skin conditions involving zinc deficiency.

In late 1982 the University of California-Davis School of Veterinary Medicine took the unusual measure of alerting practitioners to what it regarded as a "newly-recognized skin disease."

"During the last three months, we have recognized a skin disease in association with the consumption of various generic dry dog foods sold by a number of supermarket chains," the bulletin said.

In case you are not familiar with generic brands, these are products marketed by supermarkets that have plain labels and usually sell for much less money than the highly advertised national brands.

The Davis alert described a number of common allergy-like signs related to the new skin disease. The signs included hair loss, and red itchy and crusting skin. In addition there was fever, enlarged lymph nodes and evidence of a supressed immune system in more severe cases.

The researchers believed that the cause of the condition was a zinc deficiency. I frankly believe the problem is not zinc alone but a deficiency in other essential nutrients along with an overdose of impurities.

Buying generic products for your animals may be an invitation to trouble. Cheaper price means cheaper ingredients and inferior nutrition. That's what a 1985 University of Georgia study concluded. I should point out however that I see plenty of skin disease in animals eating top of the line as well.

There can be other factors involved in skin-related zinc problems that mimic allergies.

Dr. G. Robert Fisher, an associate of mine, treated a four-year-old female husky who seemingly evidenced the same kind of skin problems as the Davis dogs. Her name was "Tasha" and she was eating one of the top dry products on the market. She suffered from hair loss and red, itchy skin on her face and legs.

Antibiotic and steroid medication helped the situation temporarily. But in two months it was back again. Fisher suspected a zinc problem and began supplementing the animal — first with 50 milligrams of zinc sulfate daily. There was immediate response but not total improvement. A month later he upped the dosage to 200 milligrams daily and that eliminated the problem.

"Tasha" may have been an example of a zinc-related genetic condition that frequently affects Siberian Huskies, Alaskan Malamutes, Doberman Pinschers and Great Danes. Studies have shown they have a decreased capacity for zinc absorption from the intestines. The ensuing deficiency often shows up in the form of a skin condition. It seems to respond quite well to mega zinc supplementation.

Kittens lacking proper zinc in their diets can suffer from poor hair coats, scaly and ulcerating skin. Again, supplementation is an effective remedy.

OTHER DEFICIENCY PROBLEMS

There are other ways to account for mineral deficiencies:

● Do you feed your pet cow's milk? Research has shown that milk can interfere with calcium, the very mineral it is so highly touted to provide. "Fatty acids in whole cow's milk form insoluble soaps with calcium in the intestine and slip out in the form of fatty, malodorous stools before calcium can be absorbed," according to Prevention Magazine's "Complete Book of Minerals for Health."

Earlier I mentioned that milk is highly allergenic. It will often produce an intestinal turbulence that can effectively reduce the intake of nutrients.

● One other commonly recognized depleter of calcium is too much protein. The excess actually speeds up the intake of calcium. But the kidneys panic at the sight of all this calcium and channel it out through the urine before it can go to work in the bones and other tissue where it is needed.

The drain on calcium may in fact contribute to an osteoporosis condition in older animals, particularly among cats. We find many geriatric cats with weak, brittle and decalcified bones. This can also occur among young animals who are fed predominantly meat diets. Meat has an extremely high phosphorus-to-calcium ratio, something like 20-1. Both minerals are needed to build strong bones. But too much phosphorus in the diet and not enough calcium, can create brittle bones. I have treated many growing Siamese kittens so severely decalcified that they would sustain leg fractures during normal activities.

A product such as high-protein kibble may be double trouble. The protein may promote calcium excretion. It may also irritate the stomach and intestines, creating an inflammation that hampers digestion and absorption of nutrients.

● The impurities widely present in many food products can also cause intestinal irritation and interference with nutrient absorption.

● Many animal owners are oil happy. The second they spot a dry, scaly skin, out comes the bottle of vegetable oil to be added to the daily diet. It's also popular to use oil as a coat conditioner — to create those rich, glistening coats. Well, you may be doing your animal more harm than good.

Feeding that extra oil may coat the intestinal lining and prevent uptake of water soluble vitamins and essential minerals, particularly calcium and phosphorus. I have seen many oil-supplemented puppies with signs of rickets — limping, loss of bone structure and apparent pain — even though they were receiving extra calcium. The oil was blocking calcium absorption.

Veterinarians will often recommend oil as a remedy for a constipated animal. The idea is that you coat the intestines to prevent the uptake of water. Results: loose stools. This may be OK for short-term therapy, but oil over the long haul will block nutrient uptake and cause problems. You may want to create loose bowels for a constipated animal but you surely don't want to create diarrhea in a healthy animal. And feeding it extra oil often does just that.

● Certain small breeds of dogs, namely Pomeranians, Teacup Poodles, and Shelties, frequently develop a condition in which there is an impaired ability to store sugar in the liver. In order to keep blood sugar at normal functioning levels, such animals have to be fed syrup or honey. Too much of the sweet stuff, however, can cause water to be drawn into the intestines, resulting in swelling and interference with the uptake of minerals.

7

The Enzyme Connection

"Boss" is the star of the Beverly Hills Police Department's Canine Corps. He is a highly-trained German Shepherd who has helped apprehend over 50 criminals and twice won the gold medal as the outstanding police dog in California.

However, for the longest time, "Boss" was a source of great concern for his handler, Officer Jay Broyles.

I first saw the dog in 1984. Broyles brought him in for an examination and told me the following story:

"Each year in California the top animals compete in a 'Police Dog Olympics.' The competition includes obedience tests, obstacle courses, speed drills and attack skills. 'Boss' won in 1982, the first time we entered him. That was shortly after we got him from Germany. He was outstanding.

"But inside of a year he developed a lameness in his legs that would return from time to time. Unexpectedly, during some vigorous activity, he would abruptly stop, pull up lame and go down in obvious agony. It might come after jumping a barrier during a training session or just chasing a ball in the backyard. He would be laid up and lame for four to six weeks after each episode.

"The veterinarian we consulted diagnosed the problem as pan-osteitis (a bone disease that strikes puppies). The diagnosis was puzzling because the dog was already over three years old, a mature adult. The veterinarian prescribed a cortisone medication and said the dog would outgrow the condition. But he didn't.

"'Boss' would have a couple of incidents like this every year. Luckily, it never happened on the job. He has always performed marvelously. But there has always been a nagging bit of fear in the back of my mind that something could happen at a critical moment.

"We obtained 'Boss' when he was two-years-old and he has worked with me and lived with our family ever since. Once he saved my life by attacking an armed suspect who would otherwise have shot me if 'Boss' hadn't gotten to him. Obviously we are very attached to him. We are very concerned about losing this great animal."

Officer Broyles came to see me for a second opinion. He told me about the pan-osteitis diagnosis which is extremely rare in adult dogs.

I examined "Boss" and found a chronic skin disorder on his back, underside and heels. I took a stool sample and tested for trypsin deficiency. Trypsin is one of the digestive enzymes produced by the pancreas.

I suggested taking the animal off the commercial brand of dry food he was eating and prescribed a hypoallergenic diet. I thought this might help with what looked to me like a typical food-related skin allergy.

The tests showed that "Boss" was deficient in trypsin. This deficiency was probably affecting nutrient absorption, including calcium and other minerals vital for the strength of bone tissue. He apparently was not able to keep his bones properly mineralized and that was causing the pain and lameness.

The therapy included diet change and supplementation with enzymes and calcium. "Boss" responded dramatically to the program and in less than two months he appeared to be his old tough guy self again. The pain and lameness has not recurred.

The animal's skin problem also cleared up rather quickly. The hair coat began to glow. And he even gained weight. Broyles said the dog was more alert than ever.

"Boss" improved to such a degree that it was decided to enter him in the 1985 "Police Dog Olympics." He hadn't competed since 1982 because of his condition.

An elated Officer Broyles called me to report that "Boss" did it again. He beat out 49 other dogs — the cream of California's canine cops — to win the gold medal. And a few months later he outperformed 32 other dogs to win the first ever "Police and Fire World Olympics."

SHORT ON ENZYMES, LONG ON TROUBLE

The key to "Boss's" problem was trypsin, a generally overlooked enzyme vital to the health of man, dog and cat. It is one of the digestive enzymes produced in the pancreas and secreted into the small intestine upon the arrival of food. Long thought to be mainly involved with protein, recent research has shown than trypsin's biggest contribution is breakdown of fats and carbohydrates.

The classic sign of severe trypsin deficiency is an animal eating its own stool. In the absence of adequate trypsin, food passes through the gut without nutrients being properly extracted and dispatched into the bloodstream for use in the body. In this situation, an animal instinctively eats large volumes of food to feed the crying demand for nourishment, then passes large stools containing much undigested matter, and then frequently re-ingests the stool because the nutritional demand still hasn't been met. Such animals are usually very thin and eat insatiably.

In the gut a trypsin deficiency can contribute to the same kind of chaos I have related elsewhere in the book to other causes. In this case, the poor breakdown of fats and carbohydrates creates further logjams, irritation and inflammation. The animal overloads with food. Intestinal traffic clogs with food that is poorly processed and absorbed.

"Boss" wasn't producing enough trypsin to adequately process his food and extract the vital nutrients a working dog needs to stay fit. It wasn't a severe deficiency but bad enough in his case to cause serious problems.

In my clinical research I find many animals with minor or moderate degrees of this enzyme deficiency. Even if not severe, this results in malabsorption and problems. The impact on health can show up early in kittens or puppies or possibly take several years. Often there is an allergic-like dermatitis, hair loss, and red, scaly itchy skin that an animal constantly gnaws on. In rapidly growing puppies, hunting and working dogs, there is often an accompanying lameness. "Boss" was a prime example. He had both the skin condition and the lameness.

Imagine the potential for trouble if you have a working animal or a fast-growing puppy with a trypsin deficiency. Both animals are under heavy stress and need maximum nutrition. Add a high-protein diet and you invariably make the situation worse — more intestinal chaos, less nutrient absorption. Add an oily coat condition and that's even more fuel on the flames.

One notable case I had involved a Rotweiler puppy. His owner brought him in for a skin condition, weight loss and a rotating lameness of the legs. The dog was eating a high-protein kibble, getting a daily dose of coat conditioner and, just to top it off, a hardy serving of milk. The owner wanted to make sure the growing dog was receiving enough calcium.

The road to hell, they say, is paved with good intentions. This poor dog, the recipient of the best intentions, was clearly in hell. To start with he had a mild trypsin deficiency. The owner compounded the problem, first with kibble, then with the coat conditioner and then with milk, a leading allergen. The dog suffered intestinal fire and brimstone and was sorely lacking in nutrition.

I cut out the high-protein, the coat conditioner and the milk and put him on a hypoallergenic diet. I also started him on an enzyme supplement. In one week he was greatly improved. In a short period of time his skin and lameness problems cleared up and he began putting on weight again.

This kind of moderate deficiency is also common in cats. They will manifest dermatitis plus a variety of little chronic disorders. They will eat more than usual but still look thin and unhealthy.

In three generations of one Abyssinian line I found similar problems of generalized dermatitis, weight loss and lethargy. A genetic trypsin deficiency had been passed on from grandfather to father to son. In each case, by one year of age the cats began to develop dry, brittle and coarse hair coats, itching, and start to lose weight. With an enzyme supplement all returned to full health and vigor.

In the past, chronic diarrhea in young kittens has usually related to improper diet or parasites. Over the years I have frequently found a trypsin deficiency involved. Very often there is a combination of all these things.

A small, slow-growing kitten — or puppy — may be the sign of an enzyme deficiency that is retarding normal development.

I find this situation so prevalent that every animal who enters my clinic is routinely tested for trypsin along with the usual test for parasites. This procedure has yielded a startling statistic: nearly a quarter of the animals who pass through here have small or moderate trypsin deficiency.

In my experience the mild cases of trypsin deficiency vastly outnumber the severe cases. The obvious tell-tale signs usually associated with severe deficiency may therefore not be present. Instead, the problems that manifest seem to represent other causes. Mild trypsin deficiency is largely overlooked in veterinary medicine. I believe this should be corrected. I suggest that testing for trypsin may provide the answer to many cases that defy solution.

The causes for trypsin deficiency may be two-fold:

1. Genetic. I have traced it through three generations of Abbysinians and Persians in cats. In dogs, I have found it frequently among German Shepherds, Dobermans and Irish Setters. It will show up in kittens and puppies as soon as they graduate to solid food. You will see voluminous stool, often with the undigested fat clearly visible. Animals may eat their own feces. They will often be extremely thin despite ravenous appetite.

2. Acquired. Anything adversely affecting the pancreas can impair trypsin production. Viral and bacterial infections can do that. But, as we have seen earlier, so can food allergies. I believe they are frequently involved in creating chronic inflammations inside the gland that impairs both secretion channels and production tissue for pancreatic enzymes. Degeneration of the pancreas, a result of the aging process, can also interfere with enzyme activity. I find the acquired deficiency commonly among Siamese and Abbysinian cats and, among dogs, the Miniature Poodles, Miniature Schnauzers, Shitzus, and Cocker Spaniels.

MEDICATION IMPAIRMENT

An important point to keep in mind is that an animal with a trypsin deficiency may have difficulty absorbing medication as well as food. In the absence of adequate enzyme, undigested food components can clog the gut and absorption surfaces and significantly block the uptake of medication. This provides one explanation why, in many cases, oral medication is ineffective. Veterinarians often are able to obtain desired therapeutical results only when they resort to injectables. This direct method bypasses possible roadblocks in the intestines.

Later, in Chapter Sixteen, I will discuss a simple test that can be done by your veterinarian to determine the presence of trypsin deficiency. It is well worth the small cost to have it done.

8

Breeder's Blight — The Genetic Problem

The great value of cats used to be their ability to keep a granary or household free of rodents. Dogs have been cherished as the hunter's sidekick, as sentinels and loyal companions.

Domesticated animals were largely maintained for a specific purpose and they were bred — or left to breed, according to their own urges —for that purpose and function.

But animals have changed...or, to be more precise, have been redesigned by man, the amateur creator.

GOING TO THE DOGS?

For working dogs, animals with the greatest stamina, ability and intelligence have been preferred as breeding stock in an attempt to perpetuate these qualities. A husky of great beauty but no staying power would be passed over in this selective process. The overwhelming assets were performance and filling a human need.

Dogs are still bred for function but for the most part they are now bred for a fashionable look and structure, for fad and for sales.

In northern California there are still sled dog trials. The animals entered in these competitions are bred for function — for pulling, for stamina, for vigor.

But down in southern California, where I practice, the same types of dogs are bred for looks, for beauty shows, for the ribbons and titles that fetch high prices for offspring.

The breeds may be the same but the vitality and health of the working animals seem to be vastly superior to the ones bred for beauty.

Richard A. Wolters, veteran trainer and author of "Gun Dog," "Water Dog," and other popular books on hunting dogs, says that show standards and breeding for fad and sales over many generations have changed many hunting animals.

"You now have a situation where there are non-hunting, hunting breeds," he says.

"Not only have dogs lost their hunting ability (the nose), but in many cases the temperaments and coats have changed. There are probably other negative changes as well, such as to health.

"When working animals are bred, you look for the best hunters, the most vigorous animals. But if you are breeding for a look, then ability and vigor do not seem to come into the equation.

"The American Cocker Spaniel, a good hunter when I was a boy, can't hunt his way out of a paper bag now. He no longer has a hunting nose and his hunting coat is gone. He was turned into a pet and a temperamental, feisty one at that.

"The Irish Setter used to be an excellent hunter. Today, he is gorgeous, mahogany, with hair down to his ankles. But he's a big happy, vivacious idiot. He jumps gleefully about and you can't train him.

"The Black Labrador, originally a hunting dog, is now the third most popular dog in the United States. That kind of popularity spells trouble! Last century a Yellow Labrador was rare and considered a freak. Such animals were put down. In this century, they realized the yellow was a recessive gene and they started breeding for the yellow color. Now in England there are probably more yellows than blacks and they are non-hunters. They are bred for color, not for field ability. The newest Labrador fad is chocolate and there are very few decent hunters among them."

Jim Keel, of Carmel Valley, California, has owned and bred hunting dogs for many years. He is convinced there is a health and vigor difference between function and show animals.

"Among English Setters you have show dogs and field dogs and they are absolutely two different animals despite being the same breed," says Keel.

"Years ago people began breeding the classic Setters for glamour, for the dog shows. They turned the breed into large, long and lanky animals, like the Irish Setters, and not worth a damn in the field. Others, interested in the field ability of these animals, bred for speed, stamina and and kept them as they were, small and barrell-chested.

"The show Setters have long, droopy eyelids that are disastrous out in the field because of all the dirt and pollen they collect. They can't hack it. They try but they don't have the nose or the stamina anymore. And from what I have seen they definitely have more health problems. They have runny eyes. They bite at skin that's obviously irritating them, even when there are no fleas around.

"The hunting Setters seem to live longer, fifteen years or so. One of my favorite dogs, 'Sober Sam of Santa Monica,' was a good example of this stoutness. He lived and hunted until seventeen, even surviving a shotgun wound in the head at age fifteen accidentally inflicted by a hunting friend of mine. Compared to the show dogs, he was a runt, almost half their size. But what a hunter! What a runner! What a stud! What a healthy animal until the end!"

The bulldog is a prime example of what can happen when man tampers with nature. At one end, the facial skin folds and a breeder-shortened face cause chronic dermatitis and respiratory difficulties.

At the other end, there's a serious testicle problem. About fifteen years ago constant inbreeding of the English Bulldog in England was seen to be producing dogs with only one descended testicle. The undescended testicle, while maintaining full function, remained inside the body throughout an animal's life. This was clearly a genetic phenomenon.

The situation became so widespread that the English breeders changed the judging standards to accommodate the new development. Thus today in England, the one-testicled Bulldog is fully accepted. A genetic freak was created, validated, and then perpetuated.

The health consequences of this development may not easily be swept under the carpet. An undescended testicle is subjected to higher temperature because it is contained within the body cavity. This may result in a greater production of testosterone, the male hormone. This, in turn, can lead to behavioral changes and aggressiveness. By two years of age there is a 40 percent chance of a growth developing in the undescended testicle. To date, three varieties of growths have been recognized, one of which is malignant.

We are seeing more of these abnormalities in the United States but such animals are not yet accepted for showing. Nevertheless, they are still bred, which I regard as unfortunate. Why perpetuate a freak?

I know of a California veterinarian who will take English Bulldogs with the undescended testicle, give the animal certain hormones, and surgically pull down the testicle so it appears normal. Thus the dog can be shown and bred.

I vigorously condemn such practices. A cosmetic operation is performed to create a dog who looks normal. The animal is bred and the genetic flaw marches on.

Many offspring are now turning up with *both* testicles undescended. This situation can lead to sterility. Perhaps only when this happens will the breeders stop their folly.

Another example of breeding fallout involves the collies. As a student in veterinary medical school in the early 1960s we began to see collies developing multiple eye problems. It seemed to be an overnight phenomenon.

What had happened is that the natural look of the Collie — as made famous by "Lassie" — had become unfashionable. The big eyes and wide head that nature created were apparently deemed declasse by the breeders. They preferred a long, narrow face with small eyes. I don't know how long it took for natural evolution to make the Collie what he was but virtually overnight the "fashion designers" of the canine world recreated the Collie according to their own blueprints. With the change came problems. We began seeing prematurely blind dogs and dogs with detached retinas.

I remember vividly the first case we ever examined. It involved a man in the thick of the new breeding trend. He staged shows in shopping centers, putting his stable of collies through a variety of stunts. In one of the tricks the dogs would climb up a 10-foot ladder onto a tower and then jump down into his arms. One of his star dogs missed the target once, and then twice...landing both times unhurt on the ground. After the second miss the owner brought the animal to the hospital. The case was diagnosed as early retinal degeneration.

The condition became fairly widespread among Collies and Shelties and came to be known as progressive retinal atrophy. Today, breeders of these dogs submit their animals for eye examinations in order to obtain certification for breeding. This has resulted in better control of the problem. One Midwest breeder told me that the condition is largely kept alive by the unscrupulous practices of "puppy mill" operators, who turn out animals in assembly-line fashion with little or no concern for health factors.

Interestingly, in England, where there is no certification program, the "Collie Eye Anomaly," as the condition is called, is on the rise. Fully 60 to 70 percent of the collies and shelties are said to be affected there.

Scotty cramp, a defect in the central nervous system of Scottish Terriers, is another byproduct of selected breeding over generations of animals. Scotties with this condition have difficulty walking and even standing when they become excited.

Dr. Kenneth Meyers, a research veterinarian at Washington State University, has determined that a recessive gene became entrenched in the Scotties gene pool and is responsible for the cramping problem. He feels the condition can be eliminated by 1) testing puppies for the disease before sale and 2) mating only dogs who do not carry the flawed gene.

CAT-ASTROPHIES

The situation among cats is not much better.

In veterinary clinics around the country we are seeing more cardiomyopathies than ever — enlarged hearts that lead to heart failure and death. We are also seeing more hyperthyroidism, accompanied with a terrific weight loss. Such abnormalities are thought possibly to have genetic causes.

We are seeing Persians and related breeds with the chronic runny eye and nose problem, the result of man-made structural changes to the shape of the head. These changes are also causing mechanical irritation to the eyes.

They are breeding such long faces now in the Siamese that the brains and nervous systems are affected. There is a growing incidence of seizures, and, as one breeder put it, "the cats are ding-bats."

Terrible skull and facial deformities are being reported among Burmese cats. According to a May 1982 article in Veterinary Medicine/Small Animal Clinician, more than 100 cases of grossly flawed purebred Burmese in at least thirteen widely separated states had been identified.

The authors of the article also cited a number of other significant health problems among Burmese. These include a common heart disease among kittens, a herniation of the abdominal wall, skin plaques and a malabsorption problem.

A number of veterinary schools have been investigating the situation among Burmese. Suzanne Beedy, a top breeder in San Jose, participated for four years in one such research program in conjunction with the University of Minnesota and Cornell University.

"There is a definite genetic defect among certain lines of Burmese resulting in monster-headed kittens," she says.

"What we learned is that those lines produced a big-headed look that was closer to the classic standard than ever before. This, for breeders, amounted to a giant leap forward, or at least so we thought.

"But when we got this spiffy show kitty we also got some horribly deformed kittens in the litter — cats with heads three times normal size, herniations of the brain through holes in the skull, grossly deformed bone tissue, missing noses, and displaced eyes.

"If you breed to these specific lines you have the potential to get litters with both beauties and the beasts, with kittens reflecting varying degrees of the defect. The defect in its extreme manifestation is deathly and in its very mild form it is close to the ideal standard. The most successful show burmese are, so to speak, very mildly defective.

"When we published the findings, we recommended that breeding to the afflicted lines be discontinued.

"Some responsible breeders suggested going back to safe lines and then slowly working with them to try and recreate the classic look. But others took a different attitude which was essentially, 'to hell with it, I want a winner and I don't care how I get it.'

"I would estimate that perhaps 30 percent of the Burmese breeders chose to disregard the indisputable evidence. They continue to breed and sell these lines of cats that will inevitably produce the defect. They proliferate the problem.

"This defect was once exclusive to Burmese. No longer. It has spread to certain lines of Tonkinese (Burmese and Siamese crosses) and Bombays (Black American shorthair and Burmese crosses). And it has spread from America to Europe among pure Burmese. When people are irresponsible, how can you stop such a thing? You can't."

Beedy became so discouraged with the practices among certain Burmese breeders that she chucked in 10 years of working with Burmese and switched to Abyssinians.

"There is a real problem being caused by an increase among uninformed individuals calling themselves breeders," she adds. "Such people typically will buy a registered female cat and the next minute call themselves breeders. They have no experience. No education. No awareness of the problems. Unfortunately, these individuals do a great deal of damage. They offset the good work of the many sincere and responsible breeders, people with experience, knowledge and integrity who attempt to provide the pet buying public with the personality and looks that are sought while at the same time seeking to produce as healthy an animal as possible.''

Laneen Firth, also of San Jose, is a leading breeder of grandchampion Persians. She is outraged over some of the current breeding practices.

''Sure, they may be creating some gorgeous animals, but en route they are also creating a lot of monsters and animals who have no health and no longevity,'' she says.

''Today there is just too much close inbreeding, the result of too many breeders unwilling to maintain an adequate stock of animals. They breed mother-son, father-daughter, sister-brother, etc. And they are producing problems from nose to tail.

''I don't breed any closer than aunt to nephew, uncle to niece. I don't double. I don't breed half-brothers or half-sisters, etc.

''As you set in the type for the show bench, if you double in that gene you are also doubling on any fault that may exist. We see many problems from this — one undescended testicle, bad liver, heart or kidneys, gross skull and facial deformities, hip dysplasia, five or six toes on the back feet, excessive tearing of the eyes and many cats dying suddenly from 'unknown causes.'

''Some of today's breeding practices are designed simply to produce the show cat. The victims in this headlong rush for glory are monster kittens with wierd defects and kittens with chronic disabilities — both expressions of a genetic flaw. The former have no longevity, no health to survive. They are usually put to sleep. It is the latter cats that are the real problems. They are walking veterinary bills and heartache for the families that buy them.

''I am not just talking about Persians, but all breeds. Some breeders will go to a plastic surgeon to correct a defect and, if the animal lives long enough, then breed it. That's abominable. They are even doing orthodontia work on cats to cover up flaws.''

Dr. Michael W. Fox, director of the Institute for the Study of Animal Problems, is outspoken about the harm being done to animals through improper breeding practices. For sure, he says, the show standards established for many breeds are leading to genetically-related abnormalities that can result in unnecessary suffering.

Fox also takes the veterinary medical establishment to task for not demonstrating sufficient concern about animal health and welfare. If it were, he says, ''there would be far more public awareness...for the plight of purebred pets afflicted with inherited abnormalities...'' and also about the improper diets and lifestyles to which so many pets are subjected.

FASHIONABLE DEGENERATION

I have no wish to make a blanket criticism of breeders. Many are very dedicated and conscientious people who care a great deal about the health of their animals. These are people who take time to study the problems and who seek to improve all aspects of their breed. I salute these individuals and always enjoy working with them.

Unfortunately, quite a few breeders are inexperienced and unaware of health ramifications.

Then there are the operators of "puppy mills" and "kitty mills" who create sickness and problems enmasse. These businesses are deplorable.

Some breeders are "kennel blind." They tend to close their eyes to stock faults while striving single-mindedly for the titles and sales they believe a particular look or structure will bring.

"If a breeder is producing a beautiful line of animals that unfortunately has say a respiratory or allergy problem, that person may just continue turning out the line because it is attracting attention and sales," one Southern California dog breeder told me. "The health problem is ignored. Looks are by far the No. 1 consideration."

Among Dobermans there is a fairly prevalent condition called Von Willibrand's Disease. It is something like hemophilia among humans — uncontrolled bleeding.

I know of a breeder who blatantly shrugs off the implications of this condition and mates bleeders who in turn produce more bleeders who in turn are bred by others and they produce more bleeders. This is the way a weak line can clearly erode the vitality of a breed and proliferate disease.

The look of breeds appears to be a dynamic, changing thing, like the world of fashion. Influential show judges and breeders determine what's currently in style.

Over the last twenty-five years the "in look" among Dobermans has changed every five years or so. During the sixties a taller dog with a big masculine head, almost like a Dane, was most desirable. Then a smaller and more muscular look became vogue. Then it went tall again. Then small again, with a more refined appearance where males closely resemble females.

Breeding has largely turned down a cosmetic corridor, away from more natural or functional criteria. Animals, like our food, are becoming more and more processed, more and more unnatural, more and more unhealthy.

There is a frightening surge in allergic and serious disease running through breed and family lines and then spilling out to mixed breeds. Both in dogs and cats. I am firmly convinced that contemporary breeding practices are directly related to the disease epidemic.

I suspect that the hardy "All-American" mutt or alley cat is fast disappearing. Hybrid vigor ain't what it used to be. Random cross-breeding spreads pureblood faults. The mating of a German Shepherd with food allergies, a trypsin deficiency and dysplasia, with a Siberian Husky who has interdigital cysts and allergies, is likely to produce offspring with all those problems and more.

From what I see in my practice and from what I hear other veterinarians are experiencing, I believe the fallout from erroneous breeding practices may be reaching catastrophic proportions — a wholesale susceptibility for sickness being passed down from generation to generation.

In my clinic I have been keenly interested in one apparent consequence of fad breeding. It is an endocrine defect that undermines the immune system. I call it "the dinosaur syndrome" because I think it has the potential to wipe out the pet population. In Chapter Nine I will explain the astounding impact of this overlooked problem.

This particular genetic flaw is aggravated by the unnatural food that animals are fed today. Years ago, foods were less altered, less processed. There were few or no hormones or chemical additives in food. There were no discards, byproducts and undesirable food sources laden with toxins.

We have gone from food of greater natural biological value to food that is artificial, imbalanced and often below minimum nutritional requirements.

Furthermore, animals have been taken out of their original habitats, situated in genetically-foreign enviroments, and subjected to strange things indeed.

You find cold weather huskies in Florida and Southern California...game dogs corraled in apartments and "exercised" daily at the end of a short leash...Old English Sheepdogs with long facial hair deliberately groomed over their eyes — impairing vision and the health of their eyes —all for the sake of a fashionable look.

Cats, with a prowling and solitary hunter's temperament and once with the run of the barn, are today's pampered pets, penned up in tiny apartments for a lifetime. For the preservation of the furnishings, they are often neutered, so they won't spray, and declawed, so they won't scratch. Sometimes they belong to multiple animal households and catteries, where a phenomenon known as "social stress" can undermine their health.

All things considered, the ingredients for disease are obvious. You have major negative influences working simultaneously, feeding and aggravating each other. It's a matter of addition: emotional stress plus environmental stress plus dietary stress plus misguided breeding = trouble, lots of it.

9

The Adrenal Timebomb

The timebomb is hidden deep within the viscera. To reach it you penetrate the skin in the mid-abdominal area, then the subcutaneous fatty layer beneath. You pierce a tendonous-like band called the linea alba, which binds the stomach muscles. Then comes the peritoneum, the lining of the abdominal cavity. Inside the cavity, you come first upon the great omentum, the net-like drape of tissue that binds and protects visceral organs. Parting this thin curtain, you now see part of the stomach, the purplish spleen next to it, the deep brown liver above, and in the center, the pink intestines processing a cargo of food with an undulating rhythm.

Probing still deeper, you move this winding mass to the sides and see, one on each side of the large aorta artery and the vena cava vein, the bean-shaped kidneys. Behind them is the rib cage. In a large dog each kidney is the size of two silver dollars side-by-side, in a cat or small dog, two walnuts. And there, perched next to the inside head end of each kidney are the cream-colored, thumbnail-shaped adrenal glands.

The adrenals belong to the endocrine system, a scattering of glands throughout the body that secrete minute but powerful amounts of chemical substances which have specific effects on other organs and parts.

Within the outer section of the adrenals — called the cortex — is the focus of our attention. We are primarily interested in the middle layer of the cortex. This part of the gland is not as celebrated as the inner cortical layer where the sex hormones estrogen and androgen are produced nor as well known as the other half of the adrenal — called the medulla — where adrenalin is made.

Yet, as you will see, the middle layer is very important. It delivers cortisol to the body.

Cortisol is the hormone regulating the activity of the white blood cells known as lymphocytes, the immune system soldiers that produce antibodies to fight off virus, bacteria, disease and toxic matter.

The cortisol, in turn, is regulated by a hormone produced by the pituitary gland. This hormone, called adrenocorticotropin or ACTH for short, prods the adrenal gland into production when cortisol levels are too low and applies the brakes when there's too much circulating cortisol.

Thus, there is a finely tuned feedback system between the pituitary and adrenal glands of the endocrine system that directs a major arm of the body's defense network.

When this system is in normal balance the white blood cells naturally recognize the difference between friend and foe. They turn their chemical weapons on the enemy. They don't attack the healthy tissue of the host body.

That's the way it should be and, for the most part, used to be. Until man, it appears, got into the act.

By bending the looks and structure of various breeds to meet artificial cosmetic standards, man has apparently put a kink into the genetic chain and inflicted heavy damage to canine and feline health.

After fifteen years of clinical investigation, I am convinced that the critical regulating mechanism linking the endocrine and the immune systems has been seriously damaged by excessive cosmetic breeding.

Simply put, the middle layer of the adrenal cortex, that endocrine "micro-chip," is defective. And the end result of this genetic defect, as it is passed down from generation to generation, from purebreds to purebreds, from purebreds to mixed breeds, and from mixed breed carriers to other mixed breeds, may be the proliferation of animals increasingly programmed for self-destruction. Specifically why the cortisol mechanism has been affected I don't know. That will take genetic investigators to sort out.

Early on in my practice of veterinary medicine, I became thoroughly perplexed by the constant confrontation of end diseases that no one had answers for. Neither the textbooks nor continuing education classes nor more experienced veterinarians could explain or provide solutions for the influx of allergic conditions and terrible afflictions I was seeing in both young and old animals. Seemingly at every turn I encountered severe hypersensitivity, skin with widespread inflammation, ulcerations and itchiness, chronic vomiting and diarrhea, generalized mange, internal systems out of control, and dying animals. Moreover, I was often finding similar problems among littermates and along familial lines. I began to suspect a genetic problem.

For many of these conditions, veterinary medicine commonly relies on a family of cortisone-based drugs (steroids), which are synthetic replicas of cortisol. They are anti-inflammatory and anti-itching agents that usually work with great efficiency for a certain period of time.

Varieties of these cortisone drugs are widely and intensely used by the medical profession — both for humans and animals. The possibility occurred to me that maybe we might be supplying an ingredient that was somehow missing due to some unexplained — or at least unknown to me — genetic disarray. Since cortisone is an adrenal hormone replacement I started to look at the adrenal glands.

GROPING THROUGH THE BIOCHEMICAL MAZE

During some two hundred or so routine autopsies on predominantly purebred animals I removed and carefully examined the adrenals. In most cases I found adrenal cortices that were visably smaller than normal to the naked eye.

Looking at the glands under the microscope, I found grossly underdeveloped tissue. There was a lack of cellular content and structure, no matter what age — puppies, kittens, mature animals. There was often inflamed and hemorrhaged adrenal tissue.

So frequently did I find poorly developed cortices that I began to believe indeed a genetic mutation was involved.

For a number of years, veterinary pathologists have noted the existence of varying degrees of abnormal tissue — but unrelated to classic adrenal diseases and never directly linked to any signs of illness.

In man, some evidence suggests these kind of tissue irregularities may result from bacterial infections, prolonged steroid therapy, or an immunological reaction directed against the adrenal glands. This latter possibility is referred to as an auto-immune condition. The body's own protective agents turn on the body itself. Certain adrenal cortical diseases in man are thought to be auto-immune. The syndrome tends to be familial and linked to a recessive gene.

In 1978, I investigated adrenal pathology with Edwin Howard, the chief Los Angeles County Veterinary Pathologist, on several cases of severely diseased animals. One of the cases involved a six-month-old male Irish Setter with a generalized mange and skin condition. Pathologic examination indicated auto-immune adrenal destruction — a lethal attack against what was apparently genetically-defective tissue.

Not all of the autopsies I did showed such adrenal damage. Some glands appeared normal. But the animals had been profoundly diseased. I wondered then if the cortisol was biochemically flawed in some way and had contributed to sickness.

This was an important question needing an answer — whether the gland appeared defective or not, was the cortisol effective?

I conducted a simple blood test to find out how much cortisol was available. The results amazed me. In hundreds of sick animals the cortisol levels were inadequate, below normal.

That led to another question. What did this shortage mean to the system? If there was not enough cortisol controlling the lymphocytes, could they then react unpredictably to foreign stimuli, secreting maybe too much or too little antibody? Working closely with a laboratory, I developed a test to measure the secretion of the antibodies, those fighting proteins known scientifically as immunoglobulins. When the new test was conducted I found in many instances that antibody levels were either too high or too low.

The specific antibodies I checked were IgA (Immunoglobulin A), IgM and

IgG. Let's put each one in its place.

● IgA, for our discussion, is basically produced by the lymphocytes in the mucous membranes of the body. Thus it is most abundantly found in the gastro-intestinal, respiratory and urinary tracts. It is responsible for protecting these territories by neutralizing foreign invaders.

● IgM is a primitive antibody released in the blood that acts as a roadblock to slow down viruses, bacteria, and other foreign matter when they are detected in the bloodstream. This is a first line of defense.

● IgG is a secondary, more sophisticated soldier. Imagine a SWAT team. These guys have specialized biochemical weapons to neutralize specific foreign invaders.

In my continuing investigation I tested a number of sick puppies and found them to have a deficiency of both cortisol and antibodies. I gave the animals cortisone medication and found, to my surprise, that the antibody levels increased. This was totally unexpected because modern medical thinking says cortisone suppresses the immune system and should thus lower the antibody count.

What was going on? Something else was exerting an influence here. What was it?

I went back to the books and the research. The pituitary was stimulating the adrenal glands, right? But there wasn't enough cortisol being produced because the cortisol mechanism was somehow flawed. That meant there might not be enough cortisol available to shutdown the pituitary as part of the turn on-turn off arrangement between the pituitary and adrenals. Did that make sense, Plechner? I asked myself. And if so what does all that extra ACTH do if the pituitary hormone tap isn't turned off?

What I learned is that there is another part of the adrenal cortex that is responsive to ACTH — the inner layer, from whence comes the sex hormones estrogen and androgen.

If the middle layer can't produce enough cortisol to turn off the ACTH, might not the uncontrolled ACTH stimulate an excess secretion of the sex hormones? *

So I had the lab develop a test for estrogen. I then found many animals with very high levels of adrenal estrogen and some with very low levels. I learned that both irregularities mean trouble. Examples:

● 1. Too much estrogen, as with histamine, can cause tiny blood vessels to become more permeable. This allows for blood components to spill into adjacent tissue and cause inflammation and irritation.

---

* I have not found androgen to influence the conditions I am concerned about. It is interesting to note, however, that an excess of androgen is often associated with canine nymphomania. This is a situation where a female dog acts like a male and mounts other animals.

● 2. Too much estrogen also has a turn-on effect on the ''boss'' of the pituitary, the hypothalamus gland up in the brain. A new substance, called the cortico releasing factor, is then squirted into the picture. It makes the pituitary produce more ACTH, which in turn stimulates more estrogen. Here is clearly a vicious cycle.

● 3. Too much estrogen also suppresses the activity of lymphocytes and antibodies in the immune system.

● 4. Excess estrogen binds and inactivates thyroid hormone, a secretion that is tremendously vital to good health. It regulates bodily heat, metabolism and conversion of energy.

Often, a veterinarian will not be aware of the estrogen connection in animals showing what appears to be classic signs of low thyroid. The signs are obesity, loss of hair, and sluggishness. The veterinarian will test the amount of thyroid hormone in the blood and find it is normal and then go on looking for some other cause.

But some veterinarians, even though the blood tests are normal, will still act on the signs and administer thyroid hormone replacement anyway and obtain excellent results.

What has happened is that the estrogen binds the thyroid hormone, impairing its function throughout the body. The signs of low thyroid then appear. However, the blood tests show the thyroid hormone present in normal amounts. It does not tell the whole story though: the hormone is present but has been rendered inactive.

Outside of the classic hypothyroid signs, this blockage can have a subtle effect on immune function. It can alter the ability of the lymphocytes to respond normally to stimuli, thus resulting in some degree of reduced disease protection.

● 5. Meanwhile, our old friend cortisol is also highly vulnerable to any rush of estrogen. First of all, in affected animals cortisol is deficient or defective. An excess of estrogen has the ability to tie up cortisol and make it unusable; the same effect that it has on thyroid hormone. So whatever little cortisol the flawed system is producing it is now being neutralized by this out-of-whack endocrine system.

● 6. Abnormally low estrogen level, which I found in some animals, suggests to me a genetic defect not only in the middle layer of the adrenal cortex, where the cortisol is produced, but also in the inner layer, where estrogen is made. Under the microscope, I often found abnormalities in this layer, too. And just as too much estrogen neutralizes thyroid function, abnormally low production can affect it the same way. The thyroid hormone is there but the body can't use it.

You may be wondering where estrogen produced in the ovaries fits into all this. I have been talking about adrenal estrogen, produced in both male and female animals. Ovarian estrogen is found only in the females of the species and is used primarily to create an environment in the womb that is suitable for the fertilization, implantation and nutrition of the early embryos. Adrenal estrogen is more closely involved in hormonal interrelations and immune functions throughout the body.

THE CORTISONE CONNECTION

As I struggled to unscramble all these biochemical knots, I learned why cortisones (steroid drugs) were creating healthy antibody levels instead of suppressing them as would be expected.

My discovery was this: In those animals with genetically-damaged middle layer adrenal cortices, cortisone administration makes up for shortages of natural cortisol. The cortisone slows down and normalizes the production of ACTH in the pituitary, as would happen under conditions of adequate cortisol. This in turn moderates the adrenal production of estrogen.

Too much estrogen, among other things, can suppress antibody activity. Now, with cortisone substituting for cortisol and the estrogen stabilized, a better biochemical environment is created wherein the lymphocytes and antibodies can resume normal operations.

In short, the steroid treatment stops the excess ACTH, which stops the excess adrenal estrogen, which normalizes immune function. The production of ovarian estrogen is not affected.

Most veterinarians use steroids to treat a multitude of conditions. They are probably unaware that they are simultaneously correcting a cortisol deficiency — the hidden cause of the problem.

In animals with healthy adrenals, cortisone medication can indeed suppress the immune system because too much of this substance —natural and synthetic — is then present in the body. This is why treatment with cortisone often has no long-lasting benefits and leads to side-effects. In an animal with defective adrenals, the cortisone does wonders. It's a totally different ballgame.

Later, in Chapter Seventeen, I detail a precise treatment program for hormonal replacement. The information is primarily for the professional, with suggestion on how to utilize steroids for maximum health benefits without side effects.

THE "DOMINO EFFECT"

But let's get back to our original "home-grown" cortisol, made in the adrenals. As we've seen, this hormone can be ineffective, insufficient and unusable due to underdeveloped glands, interrelated hormonal disturbances or adrenal wear-and-tear from aging. Whatever the background, the cortisol is a "dud" substance. It exerts little or no regulatory effect on the lymphocytes. Uninhibited, unchaperoned, out of control, these primary protectors react erratically, producing either too much or too little antibodies.

Either extreme means trouble. Too many antibodies will attack foreign matter, as they are programmed to do, but they can also swarm into healthy tissue and begin devouring that as well. The immune system, in effect, is turning on the body it is designed to protect.

The state of too few antibodies, on the other hand, allows foreign microorganisms and toxins to gain a foothold and create damage and disease. In either case the body has lost its protection and is vulnerable to destruction.

There are many possible combinations for malfunction and disease because there are many possible combinations of endocrine-immune imbalance. The following chart shows at a glance the most common imbalance sequences — "domino effects," if you will — that I see in my practice. All originate from the defective adrenal cortex middle layer where cortisol is produced.

The chart readily indicates the vulnerability of animals with flawed endocrine-immune systems. The defect helps explain susceptibility to multiple allergies, epileptic seizures, altered behavior and why animals have minimum resistance to viruses and bacteria.

DOGS
● 1. Males and females with defective middle layer alone.
Too much ACTH ► Too much estrogen ► Ties up existing cortisol plus thyroid hormone ► Abnormal lymphocyte/antibody activity. Results: Allergies, auto-immunity, generalized demodectic mange, interdigital cysts, lick granuloma, epilepsy and abnormal behavior, chronic virus and bacterial infections.
● 2. Unspayed females with defective middle layer alone.
Too much ACTH ► Too much estrogen ► Ties up existing cortisol plus thyroid hormone. Results: Same as above, plus false pregnancies, cystic ovaries, pyometra (a severe hormonally-based uterine infection), and mammary tumors.
● 3. Spayed females with both defective middle (cortisol) and inner (estrogen) layers.
Too much ACTH ► Too little estrogen ► Blocks thyroid hormone utilization ► Abnormal lymphocyte/antibody activity. Results: Allergies, auto-immunity, epilepsy and abnormal behavior, viral and bacterial infections, urinary incontinence.

CATS
● 1. Males and females with defective middle layer alone.
Too much ACTH ► Too much estrogen ► Ties up existing cortisol plus thyroid hormone ► Abnormal lymphocyte/antibody activity. Results: Allergies, auto-immunity, milliary dermatitis, feline acne, eosinophilic granuloma, leukemia, infectious peritonitis, and feline urologic syndrome (FUS).

The cortisol defect relates to a breakdown of intestinal wall protection, where the IgA is being over or underproduced. This allows chemical toxins, insulting food molecules, and harmful germs to readily gain entry into the bloodstream.

In cats I find the cortisol imbalance related to urinary stones, the terrible gum inflammations and infections leading to loss of teeth at an early age, and to feline leukemia and infectious peritonitis. The understanding of the endocrine-immune relationship helps me provide aid to these animals.

Here are animals who have been rendered genetic cripples, walking time-bombs. The greater their adrenal damage, the greater their vulnerability to the stresses, contaminants and germs coming their way. The more they are bred for their looks the greater this disease epidemic will grow, I fear, until it may well engulf all our pets in a holocaust of destruction by disease.

They, like the dinosaurs, may not survive.

The difference between a mild allergy and a complete auto-immune collapse of the body, where the defense cells no longer recognize the host tissue, may depend on the amount of damage to the middle layer of the adrenal cortex.

This is no temporary illness or something that is outgrown. This is a major and lasting genetic defect. Once the adrenal timebomb goes off, the animal will prematurely die or live out a life with chronic health problems.

It's a mystery to me is why this endocrine-immune link to disease has not been recognized by veterinary medicine at large. It could be that this phenomenon falls between the cracks of adrenal conditions our profession is more familiar with — Addison's Disease and Cushing's Syndrome.

Addison's is an acquired or genetic adrenal deficiency of a different cortical secretion that regulates sodium and potassium balance. The resulting mineral imbalance leads to vomiting, diarrhea, muscle weakness and, finally, cardiac arrest.

Cushing's involves too much cortisol production, an acquired problem. This leads to obesity, hair loss, excessive drinking and urination, and calcification of skin.

The problem I am concerned with does not affect mineral balance. And it is a cortisol deficiency, not an excess. It is a wide-ranging syndrome with subtle or gross effects on hormones and antibodies throughout the body. It stirs up so much trouble that we veterinarians are too busy treating the individual signs and diseases to see the common cause. We see the trees, but not the forest.

I have come to regard the signs and diseases as secondaries, that is, direct or indirect results of the underlying endocrine-immune defect. The secondaries are what get treated. But the defect is left untouched. And left untouched, it continues to stir up trouble. That is why so many of our therapies are partially or temporarily effective or just ineffective altogether.

I have never found this endocrine-immune mechanism reported in the veterinary literature or textbooks as I inched along in my own clinical investigation. And the connection to cosmetic breeding has not been scrutinized at all by anyone other than myself as far as I know.

In 1976 and again in 1978 and 1979 I reported my findings in veterinary journals. The veterinarians who then began to look at this problem reported that a new therapeutic avenue was opened to them.

I am hoping this book will help bring renewed attention to the problem. It desperately needs it. Otherwise the timebomb will continue to tick away and explode and our animals continue to be programmed for suffering. Our greatest treatment for this pervasive condition lies first in recognizing its existence and secondly, in acting to prevent it.

10

When The Timebomb Explodes (dogs)

The timebomb spares no breed. From what I see, they all have it. Some more. Some less. I have found the adrenal defect in animals from all parts of the world, from the most aristocratic to the most humble of origins.

The following are selected cases, conditions and patterns of disease which have made a vivid impression on me. Obviously, there is not room to mention every breed or disease with an associated cortisol problem.

These observations are based on the specific traffic that has passed through my clinic. After many thousands of cases I feel they represent a genuine epidemic of cortisol-related problems in animals.

EXAMPLE NO. 1 — DOBERMAN PINSCHERS

"Blue Dobie Syndrome" is a serious set of problems commonly and most severely affecting a popular branch of the Doberman family. However, all types of Dobermans — Blacks, Reds and Fawns — are involved as well. I am inundated with sick Dobermans in my practice.

Trouble often starts after a few weeks of age, beginning with hair loss on the head, elbows and hocks. This condition is so commonplace that it is virtually expected with Dobie puppies — a pathetic rite of passage.

In 1979 I published a report on the genetic problem inherent with this breed. A one-year-old dark Blue female Doberman had been brought to my office. She suffered from inflamed skin and purulent sores, generalized demodectic mange, hair loss and scratching. I tested the dog and found a pronounced adrenal suppression. I recommended she not be bred because of the possibility of passing on the adrenal defect. During the treatment period, the owner even promised to spay the dog.

However, six months later the bitch was bred. The sire was a three-year-old black Doberman with a history of summer hypersensitivity dermatitis. The pregnancy was normal. The litter contained thirteen puppies.

At three weeks, all puppies developed inflamed skin and sores on the face and extremities. At twelve weeks, the signs of inherited immune disease were fully apparent. The pups had mange, severe oozing sores, swollen lymph glands and widespread inflammation.

One of the puppies was brought in for diagnostic procedures and was found to have biochemical markers similar to his mother — evidence that the offspring inherited a defective adrenal cortex. Due to the severity of the disorder, the owner requested that the puppy be euthanized. The pathology report provided by the Los Angeles County Veterinary Services indicated underdevelopment and degeneration of both adrenal cortices.

I once closely studied the biochemical profiles of several generations — a total of five animals — in one line of Blacks, supposedly the most robust of the breed. Here too I found evidence of a perpetuated adrenal defect. The majority were not only cortisol deficient, but they were also hypothyroid, had estrogen and antibody imbalances, and a trypsin deficiency.

Often by the time such dogs become sexually mature, you can see the surface signs of food allergies and progressive disorder, things such as chronic skin problems, generalized mange, ear mites, severe weight loss. These dogs often die prematurely from kidney, liver or pancreatic disease. With severe genetic damage the timebomb can explode in five or six weeks. Or it can tick away for years, causing chronic unwellness, until finally the animal dies from the failure of an essential organ.

An example of this involved a Doberman Black male who suddenly became aggressive — lunging and snapping at members of the household. The dog was about to be sent away for training but first the owners brought him in for an examination.

I did a full workup and found a cortisol deficiency, high antibodies and extremely high nitrogen in the blood. The latter is indicative of kidney trouble. I felt the dog was experiencing kidney failure with a resultant interference in normal behavior. You might call it a ''nitrogen narcosis.'' He would become disoriented and not recognize his owners.

Indeed, the kidney damage in this case was so severe that the dog had to be euthanized.

I frequently see such IgA-cortisol-related end diseases of key organs. The IgA guarding the mucous linings of these organs run wild and begin devouring healthy adjacent tissue. In the kidneys, this situation, combined with the overwork demanded by high protein diets, can lead to premature death.

The Doberman breed is also afflicted with a ligamental weakness in the neck, called the ''wobbler syndrome,'' widespread hip dysplasia, and a blood clotting problem called Von Willibrand's Disease. These ailments occur as a result of indiscriminate breeding. Increasingly, certification is being demanded by purchasers that animals are healthy and free of such disorders. I feel that this protective action should also include endocrine-immune certification.

EXAMPLE NO. 2 — COCKER AND SPRINGER SPANIELS

I hear many reports of behavioral problems as these breeds become further bred away from their traditional hunting and field functions.

One Springer Spaniel, a show animal, was brought to me by his owner who said the creature was attacking the judges at dog shows. Obviously you don't win ribbons that way. I did a workup and found a cortisol imbalance with high estrogen. The dog probably wasn't feeling well. He certainly wasn't behaving well. After identifying the problem we initiated a special diet with appropriate hormonal replacement. We were able to eliminate the anti-social behavior so the dog could be shown again.

Another case involved a Springer Spaniel I had been treating ever since he was a puppy. His initial problem was food allergies with diarrhea. It was a clear cortisol deficiency. He was subsequently maintained on hypoallergenic diets with hormonal replacement and seemed to be doing well.

When he was six years old, he was in for a checkup and a grooming session. The owner asked me to examine the dog's eyes. When I got close the dog snapped and just about took my thumb off. I told this to the owner and she said, yes, the dog had been acting bizarre at times. I did a workup and found his IgA-estrogen levels were off. The aggressive behavior reflected a deterioration of this imbalance despite our efforts to control it. The dog had become a fear biter.

In a 1984 veterinary journal article, Dr. R.A. Mugford, a British veterinarian, wrote that the frequent aggressive behavior of the English Cocker Spaniel probably has a genetic basis.

"English Cocker Spaniels have a long-established reputation for their unreliable temperament: individuals may be exceptionally excitable, moody and aggressive," and many owners ask a veterinary surgeon to euthanize their animals as a result, he said. The disturbed behavior is variously referred to as "Cocker rage syndrome" or "low threshold aggression."

Among fifty problem Cockers brought in by owners, Mugford said that 74 percent of them were Red/Golden variants, "significantly more inbred" than the particolored Cockers. In 76 percent of the cases, the dogs had displayed aggression towards their owners, 63 percent had bitten their owners, and 23 percent had bitten children in the household.

The majority of Cockers make successful "if rather excitable companions," however, an unknown proportion of them are prone to unpredictable and aggressive behavior, the British veterinarian said.

EXAMPLE NO. 3 — COCKERS, BEAGLES, STANDARD POODLES

Another common problem among Cockers is chronic ear infections. Beagles and Standard Poodles get them often as well. All these dogs have been bred away from their traditional hunting roles.

For years the infections have been attributed to long ears hanging down flat against the side of the head and thus preventing air circulation. Lack of ventilation creates a fertile bed for germs, so it is thought.

In my opinion, this is not the reason. There are many breeds of dogs with similar ear structures but without the problem. The breeds I have cited here — and add Springer Spaniels to them — seem to commonly have an IgA imbalance and food allergies. The allergies impact in the ear area where there is an abundance of histamine-producing mast cells. When the biochemical imbalances are identified, corrected and the animals placed on hypoallergenic diets, recurrent ear infections can be usually prevented.

EXAMPLE NO. 4 — DOG GUIDES FOR THE BLIND

Over the years I have treated a number of these animals, mostly Golden Retrievers obtained from a California facility that breeds and trains them.

Problems are basically similar: food allergies, gross skin conditions and abnormal behavior. It often requires specialized diet, medication and hormonal replacement to keep these animals in a functional state. Some are so seriously defective there is no way they can handle their responsibilities.

One such case was "Edson," a Golden Retriever owned by Charlene Hunt of Santa Monica. The dog was obtained at the age of one-and-a-half and, in Charlene's own words, "he was sick most of the five years I had him."

He developed severe skin sores that sometimes required treatment twice a week. On a number of occasions, people stopped Charlene in the street, absurdly accusing her of beating the dog and threatening to call the humane society. At times the sores were so bad the dog could hardly walk and Charlene would have to take a cab home from work.

"Edson" also suffered from severe diarrhea when he ate anything besides a restricted hypoallergenic diet.

Although we were able to stabilize him to some degree, he continued to decline. His energy was never good. At six-and-a-half, well before his time, he had to be put to sleep. It was a very traumatic thing for me to do. I had grown very attached to this animal and knew how much Charlene loved him.

"Edson" was the third dog she had obtained from the same California training facility. Each time the animals were unable to fulfill their responsibility. The first dog had behavior problems and was returned after three months. The second animal had hip dysplasia and food problems and needed special diets. She had to be retired early.

"I know of other guide dogs with terrible skin problems and other serious defects," Charlene says. "And when we inform the school about this they want to deny that any problems exist. That isn't right. Something should be done.

"People seem to go back to the school often, like every two years or so, for a new dog. The animals never last a good eight to ten years as they should."

Some time ago I contacted the training facility. I explained to the veterinarian there that a serious problem existed with the animals. The response was negative. My offer to help try and correct the situation was ignored.

After Charlene's negative experiences, I suggested she find another dog elsewhere. She traveled to an east coast school, hoping for better luck. There, she was assigned a German Shepherd and has had him for over a year now without any major problems.

Judy Flerman is a blind medical secretary who has been a client of mine for years. She had received a Yellow Labrador — "Haven" — who was sick from day one.

"She was vomiting practically every day while we were training together at the school," Judy recalls. "They told me she had a nervous stomach because of all the drilling and classes.

"But when we got home the vomiting continued. Two or three times a week. She was sluggish and didn't play very much. But I had grown very attached to her by then.

"For three years I took her from one veterinarian to another. It was tremendously inconvenient and expensive. It was also painful knowing she was so sick.

"A friend told me about Dr. Plechner and I took 'Haven' to see him. He was going to be my last resort. He tested her and found she needed cortisone and thyroid replacement. We started the program. That was five years ago. She's been relatively healthy ever since, kept that way on drugs and special diet.

"Today, at nine-and-a-half, she's still able to work. But the day will come soon when I will have to retire her. And I just dread the prospect of a new dog and going through this whole thing again."

The problems experienced by Charlene Hunt and Judy Flerman are repeated all over the country. They will continue until the schools stop dispensing defective dogs. I am well aware of the noble intentions of the schools. They provide animals to the blind without cost. But whether they breed the dogs themselves or accept them as gifts from generous donors, these organizations should be concerned about providing the healthiest animals they can.

As Judy Flerman says: "What's the use of all the good intentions if the dogs bring more burdens than benefits. The one thing we don't need is more burdens. We shouldn't have to bring sick dogs home. And that is happening frequently enough to make this a very unsettling business."

Clean hips and clean elbows are not enough. These animals need clean insides too. They need certification for normal adrenal cortex function, and normal antibody response. The guide dog schools should make an extra effort to ensure that their animals can serve their handicapped owners without becoming handicaps themselves.

EXAMPLE NO. 5 — LABRADORS AND GOLDEN RETRIEVERS

Black Labradors used to have that big square head and the huge tail with which to steer in water. Out hunting you would see those chunky bodies at the ready, sniffing the wind and scanning the skies. They radiated health and purpose.

Nowadays you see tall, thin, slab-sided and empty-headed labradors with their sense and function bred out of them. They run on one speed — overdrive. They are hyperactive, like yo-yos at the end of a leash.

People have tremendous difficulties trying to train them. A labrador will return from a professional trainer and the first day back he will chew up the pillows on the sofa or be carousing with the kids down the block. I hear variations on this theme all the time.

These are the the offspring of show labs. Their bloodlines may swell with champions but these animals are losers. They are out of control.

People who like this friendly breed are beginning to look for animals with field backgrounds rather than show titles. That's what I recommend. By making the distinction you have a better chance of getting a healthier and more stable animal.

"Dune," a male Golden Retriever who was ten weeks old when I first saw him, was a tough case. He was a pathetic runt when he was brought into my clinic. His body was hairless in many places. His muzzle and ears were swollen three times normal size. He was grossly deficient in cortisol and IgA and was hypothyroid.

The breeder was so upset that she brought in the bitch, an award-winning showdog. The animal had experienced only occasional mild dermatitis during the summers. Testing showed an IgA imbalance. This, her first litter, was smaller than you would normally expect.

She whelped only two puppies. We checked the other pup and he also was IgA deficient, although not hypothyroid, and apparently strong enough so far to keep the timebomb at bay.

On special diets and hormones we were able to keep "Dune" alive for six years. He was one-third the size of normal Golden Retrievers. Occasionally he would contract a harsh viral condition, indicative of an immune system still subpar despite our intense efforts. Finally, he succumbed to a pancreatic disease caused, I believe, by an IgA antibody imbalance which left the pancreatic tissue vulnerable.

Here is a case where a parent may be just somewhat off the norm. When the mate is also somewhat abnormal, the genetic flaw seems to magnify as it is passed down. And boom! you get the timebomb going off early in life with devastating effect.

EXAMPLE NO. 6 — MINIATURE AND TEACUP POODLES

The grandmother, mother and daughter of a Silver Miniature Poodle line were brought to me by their three different owners over a number of years. Each animal, until spayed, experienced false pregnancies. All had food allergies related to an imbalance of their IgA antibodies. Each was cortisol deficient with excess levels of estrogen. They suffered from chronic skin disorders, paws that would become swollen from constant biting and chewing, and itchy undersides they would scratch until blisters formed. The two younger dogs had epilepsy.

All of these animals had experienced false pregnancies and had difficulties reproducing. Each was eventually spayed. A blessing, I felt. Even if I could restore their fecundity through hormonal replacement and other therapies, the line was seriously defective. Why continue it?

I am seeing many food allergies, cystic ovaries, mammary tumors, generalized mange and, in particular, behavioral abnormalities and epilepsy in these animals.

According to the Epilepsy Institute in New York, epileptic dogs are often purebred and have a family history of the illness. It is reported to be inherited among certain breeds including Irish Setters, German Shepherds, Beagles and Poodles.

In my practice I see more epileptic Poodles than any other breed. The problem often begins when an animal is about two but it can show up anytime, earlier or later.

I am not sure, and veterinary medicine is really not sure, what creates such blow outs of the nervous system. The cause of seizures is regarded as idiopathic, that is, nobody knows precisely why they happen.

In doing workups on these cases I usually find a cortisol-IgA imbalance which is adversely impacted by foods. Additionally, there will often be a high estrogen level. This combination of biochemical imbalances and inability to process food properly may create a chronically toxic situation in the body that can eventually trigger seizures. The timebomb ticks away until one day it explodes. I have witnessed many complete remissions as a result of defusing the adrenal timebomb.

EXAMPLE NO. 7 — OLD ENGLISH SHEEPDOGS

I have found that about 40 percent of the 200 or so Sheepdogs I have attended over the years suffered from the repercussions of an endocrine-immune imbalance: gastro-intestinal disorders, skin problems, false pregnancies and epilepsy.

I closely followed five generations of one line and virtually all animals in it developed an allergy to beef after two years of age. After eating beef they would experience diarrhea, vomiting and/or an outbreak of skin problems.

Many of the affected animals become what we call "fear biters." They turn into Jekyll and Hydes. Due to a behavioral instability secondary to hormonal imbalances, they often are shy, recessive and wide-eyed in unfamiliar situations. Then out of fear they will snap and bite..and then lick you afterward.

I recall vividly one dog who bit his owner — a rock star — in the face, narrowly missing a major artery. The attack was sudden; the two had been extremely close. Here was an eight-year-old animal who had a terrible cortisol-IgA imbalance. We were able to keep him under fairly good control for years through diet and hormonal replacement. But the imbalance was too profound. After the attack he stood there and licked his master's face as if to say "Forgive me, I know not what I do."

EXAMPLE NO. 8 — BASSET HOUNDS

A ten-week-old Basset hound, the offspring of two champions, was presented in what was clearly a dying condition. Blood and serum were weeping from every pore of the body. The dog had no hair whatsoever. He was a study in misery. His sole littermate was similarly afflicted, the owner said. This was the bitch's first litter.

Tests revealed the puppy was deficient in cortisol, thyroid and antibodies. He was a sitting duck for virus and bacteria.

The parents had always experienced "acceptable" problems such as occasional hot spots and intermittent intolerance to food which manifested as flatulence, vomiting and diarrhea, the owner reported. Apparently they were fractionally cortisol deficient and passed the defect down to their progeny in whom the timebomb exploded early in life.

EXAMPLE NO. 9 — MINIATURE SCHNAUZERS

There is a recognized problem of food allergies and bladder-urinary tract infections in this breed. What probably escapes notice is the connection between both problems. On examination I constantly find imbalances of IgA. Keep in mind that IgA is supposedly protecting both the digestive and the urinary tracts.

In some animals the impact area is the gut. You will have food allergy and IgA imbalance leading to diarrhea and vomiting. Or you will have no GI reaction but instead blood in the urine. Veterinarians often have to deal with both problems concurrently.

With proper diet and adjustment of the endocrine-immune mechanism you can restore these animals back to a good life without intestinal upset, bladder problems or the tendency toward pancreatic and liver disease.

EXAMPLE NO. 10 — GERMAN SHEPHERDS

Previously the most common problem with this breed was hip dysplasia. Now I seem to be flooded with the manifestations of endocrine-immune imbalances among Shepherds.

I find many of them suffering from false pregnancies, trypsin deficiencies, food allergies, malabsorption, flea allergy dermatitis, generalized mange, ulcerative colitis, inability to gain weight, and epilepsy.

I recently treated seven Shepherds imported from Germany where they had been bred and trained for police work. The hips were clean. The elbows clean. The German breeders apparently are getting the upper hand on the dysplasia problem.

But that is only a part of the breeding problem. Each and every one of those high-powered, high-priced animals was sick in some manner. Each had a trypsin deficiency, food allergies and the endocrine-immune imbalance.

I think the breeders are going to have to recognize that the consequences of improper breeding extends beyond hips and elbows.

In this country, the popularity of Shepherds has waned over the years. I wonder if those great animals of yesteryear — the kind typified by Hollywood's "Rin-Tin-Tin" — still exist. From what I see in my practice and what other veterinarians tell me, I have my doubts.

Veterinarians nowadays are rather wary around Shepherds. Many of them are fear biters. They just aren't the gracious, solid dogs we once saw.

EXAMPLE NO. 11 — TERRIERS

I see widespread food allergies and skin conditions among the terriers, from little Yorkies all the way up to large Skyes. Often even when you correct the endocrine-immune imbalance with proper hormone replacement, many animals must be maintained on the most carefully controlled diets.

Such an example was a Kairn Terrier who almost died because her owner could not understand the seriousness of the timebomb mechanism. The dog was basically healthly while on a hormone program and a diet free of beef or chicken. She was deathly allergic to these foods.

"A little bit certainly can't hurt her," the owner kept insisting.

But a little bit could indeed hurt her. It took one exceptionally violent reaction, after a series of lesser episodes, to make the owner a believer. Just a morsel of forbidden food to this hypersensitive animal was enough to explode the timebomb.

EXAMPLE NO. 12 — MIXED BREEDS

In the old days when two healthy purebred dogs of different breeds got together and mated, the union usually produced puppies radiating with what we call hybrid vigor. The mixed blood seemed to favor and perpetuate the hardiest qualities of the parents.

But now, hardy progenitors seem to be vanishing. More often than not, today's "mixed mates" are genetically-flawed animals. When they mate, with or without man's help, they no longer seem to produce hybrid vigor. They produce amplifications of their own problems. They produce damaged goods.

A male Collie with the cortisol imbalance suffered from terrible food allergies. He was bred to the German Shepherd next door. The female had a history of false pregnancies, suffered from generalized mange and had a trypsin deficiency.

This mating produced a reduced litter of three puppies. The offspring showed little vigor, were undersized, and showed the skin signs of food allergy. I tested them at eight weeks and found they all had a trypsin deficiency.

At three months they were vaccinated for distemper. Shortly thereafter two of them died — from distemper. Obviously, their immune systems were weak and they had obviously not been unable to mount a proper response.

Do you remember "Daisy" the dog in the "Dagwood and Blondie" comic strip? She was a cockapoo — part Cocker, part Poodle.

Today, our Cockapoos are the same shaggy, sweet and lovable creatures but with little ability to flourish.

A year-old Poodle female with epilepsy and food allergies was bred to a Cocker Spaniel of three. The latter also had a history of food allergies along with premature loss of teeth and two episodes of seizures apparently triggered by a high protein diet. The result of this union was a litter of five adorable females.

But beneath the good looks there was trouble. Each of the young developed horrible false pregnancies after their first heat cycle and were spayed. Each had severe food allergies. The one I subsequently examined developed seizures by the age of two.

Do you really expect to take two genetic cripples and produce a bionic dog? Look at the problems of the purebreds I have described above. Look at their diseases. Then do some simple multiplication. Multiply the diseases of one by the diseases of the other. The result is what you may well get when you breed the two.

11

When The Timebomb Explodes (cats)

Behind much of the suffering and death of cats hides the cortisol-IgA imbalance, the genetic timebomb. It weakens the fight and fiber of animals, leaving them terribly vulnerable.

Later, in Chapter Seventeen, I discuss how to identify and defuse the timebomb. When done, this greatly enhances the ability of cats to repel the most serious threats to health.

EXAMPLE NO. 1 — FELINE LEUKEMIA (FeLV)

Have you ever wondered why some cats contract feline leukemia and most others don't?

Why is it that around 30 percent of the animals exposed to the virus actually break with it and not more?

Why is it that in a multiple cat household of unrelated animals one will come down with leukemia and not others?

My testing indicates that all cats who develop clinical signs of this very serious disease complex are adrenally-defective. They are not producing enough regulatory cortisol. The consequence is loss of lymphocyte control and abnormal antibody response to stimuli.

When the leukemia virus is encountered, these out-of-control immune systems overreact. The lymphocytes overproduce antibodies. The antibodies go on a rampage, attacking both the virus and the cat's own bodily tissue. You have a double dose of disaster: both the virus and the immune system collaborating in a destruction derby. These cats have a hormonal deficiency that is creating a hyperimmunity. If untreated, they will basically die from over-processing of the virus.

The leukemia virus can strike at almost any tissue or organ and open the door for a variety of associated diseases. Destruction takes hold depending upon how and where the virus enters the body, where it concentrates and where there may be areas of genetic weakness.

Over the years I have treated some two thousand leukemic cats, many of them terminally-ill. By applying the tests for endocrine-immune imbalance and then following-up with individualized hormonal replacement I have been able to save many of them from a probable imminent death.

"Raja," a two-year-old Burmese, was a dramatic example. Here was a cat with a severe leukemic infection attacking the kidneys. I tested him and found the classical cortisol-antibody imbalances. I carefully initiated a replacement program for his specific deficiency.

In a matter of three weeks, his previously enlarged, malfunctioning kidneys began showing signs of recovery. He was regaining appetite and vigor. Tests showed his antibodies returning to normal, meaning they were no longer devouring innocent tissue and killing the cat. At six weeks, testing indicated he was leukemia negative.

How, you may ask, is it possible that a cat with this terrible disease becomes virus-free? It is widely accepted that if the animal survives it plods on in life as a carrier, a source of potential infection for others.

But here's where the overlooked endocrine-immune mechanism comes in. You test for this defect. You find it. You correct it. You put the animal's derailed immune system on track, enabling it to fight and shed the virus just as it would any other stimulant-allergen. The cat will respond negative in testing.

I have seen this reversal many times, including even among cats with the FIP virus. Veterinary textbooks say this cannot happen. But it can if you defuse the timebomb early enough before permanent damage is inflicted to organs and vital parts. Early treatment is important.

If we had not caught "Raja" when we did, he would have suffered irreparable damage to kidney tissue. We may have been able to beat the virus but not overcome the effects of severe kidney damage.

As in this case and others, hormonal replacement therapy must be continued. If you stop it, you remove the crutch and the animal will fall. It's as simple as that. The genetic damage to the middle layer adrenal cortex is permanent. It doesn't grow back and heal itself and operate normally.

If the virus is still present and you stop the therapy, the bomb will explode again. The immune system will go haywire again. Signs of disease will return.

Even if the virus has been shed and you discontinue therapy, you are still risking the cat's health. Should the leukemia virus be encountered at a later date, immune protection would likely be inadequate.

Feline leukemia is a leading cat killer. In the scientific scramble to discover the idiosyncrasies of the virus and a vaccine to control it, no one has looked at the endocrine-immune connection. Here, I feel, is a promising avenue of both prevention and treatment. Here, perhaps, lies the cause: excessive inbreeding resulting in a genetic adrenal defect which makes the animal extra vulnerable when exposed to the virus.

"Raja" has been doing quite well since he started the replacement program more than six years ago. Interestingly, I tested one of his sons and the younger cat had the exact same cortisol imbalance. In junior's case, the timebomb was merely ticking. His antibody count was just within the normal range. The immune system was still able to elude the virus stalking this household of cats.

The timebomb hadn't exploded yet but I could see what was coming. I suggested hormonal replacement. The cat, as his father, has been on this program for several years. He has maintained normal antibodies and so far been disease-free.

Today, there is widespread interest in a new leukemia vaccine. The vaccine is a concentrate of killed leukemia viruses. After innoculation, the immune system is then expected to respond by developing the appropriate antibodies for the disease. Thus, should the real thing be encountered, the animal's immune system will be ready and primed for the fight. Or so the thinking goes.

If the cat has the genetic timebomb, the vaccine script won't work. The cortisol defect disallows normal response and buildup of antibodies. The cats who are naturally robust with strong resistance, probably won't get the disease in the first place. Their immune forces will respond and meet the attack at first sighting of the virus.

So, if you think about it, the vaccine may or may not give any added protection to the strong ones. For animals who really need the help, the vaccine probably won't be effective at all because of the adrenal weakness.

If the vaccine does any good, it may be among those intermediary cats who can resist serious infection but who cannot shed the virus. By liberating these animals, the vaccine might reduce the spread of leukemia.

EXAMPLE NO. 2 — FELINE INFECTIOUS PERITONITIS (FIP)

Up to 25 percent of the cat population is affected by this highly contagious virus. In the early stage of the disease, there is often mild sneezing with discharges from the nose or eyes. Most cats who recover from this phase nevertheless remain persistently infected and serve as carriers. If the FIP advances, it is usually fatal. There is a buildup of fluid in the abdomen and severe damage to vital organs.

As with feline leukemia, all the FIP cats I test have the adrenal defect. They tend to be hyperimmune, their bodies wildly churning out antibodies when exposed to the virus. Then, both the virus and the immune system team up to destroy the animal.

Back in 1981, I successfully treated "Mitzy," a five-year-old spayed female Domestic Shorthair. She had been declared a hopeless case by two other veterinarians. When I first saw her she was extremely emaciated, except for the bloated abdomen, and was basically dying. She had the wet form of FIP. Her abdomen was full of the typical straw-colored fluid and even her chest cavity was affected.

I treated her for the cortisol deficiency which was causing a gross overproduction of IgA. Within three weeks, she began to show signs of improvement. Her vital counts normalized. She gained weight. In two months she was negative for FIP.

I have kept her on a hormone replacement program ever since. In July 1985 she was brought in by her owner for standard vaccination. She's a big, robust and lively animal with no signs of the disease. She has been on cortisone all this time, without any side effects whatsoever. This program has kept her timebomb totally under control. It has kept her alive.

You may be surprised by my emphasis on cortisone therapy — a none-too-fashionable treatment concept. Please keep in mind that my animals are first tested. If they are found to be deficient of cortisol, the cortisone is prescribed.

Without this hormone replacement, such animals will either die or live a life of constant misery.

EXAMPLE NO. 3 — FELINE UROLOGIC SYNDROME (FUS)

FUS means painful stones and blockages of the urinary tract. If not treated, it can lead to death.

Males are more susceptible to blockage than females because of their narrower urethras, the narrow tube that carries urine out of the body from the bladder.

Regard it as a warning sign if you see a cat squatting, straining, and frequently voiding tiny amounts of urine, or if you see traces of blood in the urine. Without medical attention, poisonous wastes back up into the body, resulting in weakness, loss of appetite, vomiting and eventually death.

A combination of things cause mineral crystals, stones or plugs to form. Most commonly cited are obesity, inactivity, a high amount of magnesium in the diet, and low water intake.

Trouble occurs when small sand-like particles rub and irritate the urinary tract lining. The particles are composed of minerals and cellular slough-off and debris from the irritated lining. The particles also team up with mucoid substances to form stones that plug up the urethra.

Overlooked in all this is the cortisol-IgA imbalance. An accessory to the crime, I believe. In cases where I test animals with FUS, I often find the adrenal defect.

The lymphocytes producing IgA are present in the mucous membrane linings of the body, including the urinary tract. If an animal's imbalance swings toward too much antibody production, an overkill effect takes place. The excess antibodies attack healthy tissue in addition to foreign stimuli. This response accelerates irritation and damage to the mucous lining.

I recall a large black cat who had chronic bouts of cystitis. When he had the urge he would strain and pass little urine. The classic signs. He also had a food allergy problem which seemed to make all this worse. A blood test showed a very high IgA antibody level. I prescribed a hormone replacement program which kept him basically under control.

The cat was highly allergic to beef and I urged avoidance of any form of this food. On occasion, however, the owner would forget or not read labels and the cat would get beef. It was open sesame to pain and discomfort. Immediately the signs would return: the cat would strain, spray, act jumpy, and poke his tail up in the air with the hair on edge.

Too little IgA production can also be a problem. This results in decreased resistance to bacterial, viral and perhaps chemical substances which can aggravate the lining and feed the buildup of particulate matter.

"Kiddo," as an example, had virtually no IgA. He was a two-year-old breeding Abyssinian with a history of chronic urinary tract problems. I operated on him for removal of an acute plug and subsequently prescribed a carefully regulated diet along with hormone replacements. On this program he has been doing nicely. It keeps his genetic timebomb in check.

I have tested quite a few FUS fathers and sons and found striking similarities in their endocrine-immune imbalances. I try to keep them out of repeat trouble by closely following their food and hormone replacement programs.

EXAMPLE NO. 4 — SKIN DISEASE

Aside from flea-bite allergy, which I'll cover in the next chapter, cats are commonly plagued by three skin conditions:

● 1. Milliary dermatitis — This is a generalized, moth-eaten effect, with small scabs visible here and there on the body. Cats are miserable and may lose their appetite. They will typically take a step or two, then stop and scratch. They will often tear, lick or chew out parcels of hair. They will frequently suffer from hair balls — swallowed fur that has become impacted in the stomach.

This condition is often blamed on fleas. I don't agree. Fleas can aggravate it, but don't usually cause it.

● 2. Feline acne — Affected cats display blackhead-like growths on the chin. If the blackheads rupture internally they can cause a vicious reaction. Often the chin will swell up and mimic a cat-bite abscess or a tooth root infection.

● 3. Eosinophilic granuloma — This condition is marked by elevated, red lesions on the skin that cats will lick, bite and scratch.

In testing, cats who have any of these ailments usually present the markers of a cortisol imbalance. We veterinarians usually treat such conditions with cortisones but without the realization that there, at the heart of things, is a cortisol deficiency. More than just the expected anti-inflammatory and anti-itching effect, the cortisone is also redressing the deficiency deep down.

I believe these skin diseases follow a similar chain of events. First, the endocrine-immune imbalance causes improper processing of food or environmental toxins. The body becomes awash with contaminants and immune cells gone amok. The chaos stimulates histamine release in certain impact areas just below the skin. This creates rashes, irritation and itchiness on the surface.

Sometimes these are omens of FeLV and FIP — serious things to come if corrective measures are not taken.

EXAMPLE NO. 5 — UPPER RESPIRATORY DISEASES

These, the most widespread of feline infectious illnesses, are largely caused by viruses. Many of the infected cats I test show a cortisol-IgA imbalance. I feel this defect can create primary susceptibility in kittens and the basis for chronicity as adults. When people talk about their cats being immune-deficient and frequent prey to viruses, of suffering continual discomfort from runny eyes and runny noses, then perhaps here is the reason why.

Many cats suffer from chronic sinusitis. The frontal sinus will fill up with a heavy mucoid discharge, sometimes so severely that surgical relief is required. I have often traced this problem to irregular production of antibodies, either too little or too much.

EXAMPLE NO. 6 — GUM INFLAMMATIONS

Sometimes early, sometimes later in life, a cat may develop a bright red line along the gum line. That's a sign of inflammation which should get quick veterinary attention. Left untreated, it can lead to ulcers in the gums, recession of gum and underlying bone tissue, and finally tooth loss.

Many of the cats I have checked who have this condition also have the cortisol-IgA imbalance. Because of the defect back in the adrenal glands, there can be too little or too much IgA up front in the mucous membrane lining the mouth. Either way, food particles, bacteria, virus and other contaminants present in the oral cavity can gang up on a crippled immune system and foment irritation, infection and disease.

12

Fleas, Insects, And Inhalant Allergies

Each body — your's, mine, your pet's — has a certain capacity, or tolerance, for stress. Just how much is a matter of inheritance. The genetic blueprint sets the limits. Yours is different than the next guy's and your pet's capacity is different than your neighbor's pet.

Tolerance is like a storage tank. If you pour more stress into the tank than it can hold, it cracks, crumbles or blows up. The body breaks down.

Stress is many things: excessive physical activity, overwork, extreme cold or heat, infections, drugs, environmental and food chemicals, insecticides and pesticides, prolonged emotional disturbances, accidents, surgery, poor diet, digestive ailments that hinder absorption of nutrients, pregnancy and lactation, and hormonal imbalances.

All these elements apply to both humans and animals. Obviously, the potential for overload is high.

As far as pets are concerned, I regard four things as major problems that can shrink or exhaust capacity for stress:

● The endocrine-immune adrenal defect.
● Impure commercial pet food, stress by the mouthful.
● Mineral deficiencies.
● A trypsin deficiency.

These four factors prime an animal. They are sensitizers that create a more vulnerable and reactive cat or dog.

An animal handicapped by defective adrenal glands is going to be hyperimmune. You can expect an overreaction to environmental input.

An animal fighting the stressful ingredients of a poor diet is going to have less tolerance to fight other stresses in life.

And animals with mineral and trypsin deficiencies usually lack the nutritional building blocks their bodies need to maintain a high threshold to stress.

Onto this shaky stage steps the flea, one of the important X factors that overload the system and shatter the threshold of an animal barely coping with life. There's just no reserve with which to fight on another front.

Fleas, parasitic insects and inhalant allergens represent a seasonal assault of stress that causes breakdown and signs of allergy and disease. The casualties of this warm weather warfare then appear in droves at animal clinics everywhere.

But environmental effects can occur any time of the year. Personally, I regard all environmental allergies — the fleas, the ticks, the mites, the pollens — as secondary factors. The food, the adrenals, the minerals and the trypsin — these are the primaries. Treat them first and often you may not have to worry about the secondaries.

FLEA-ALLERGY DERMATITIS

Flea bites animal. Animal bites skin. And licks and chews and scratches ad infinitum.

It's an old story, repeated every summer. Most any pet owner knows the script by heart: loss of hair, inflamed bumps, raw, red itchy skin usually on the backside near the base of the tail, a very uncomfortable animal contorting itself to get at the itch, and ultimately a visit to the veterinarian for relief.

The entire adult life of a flea — four to six weeks on an average — is spent on the host animal. There, Dracula-like, it sucks blood to live. The adult female can deposit some twenty to twenty-eight eggs a day. Favorite depositories are animal bedding or nearby carpets, drapes and furniture. In such locations fleas rocket to maturity in about two weeks.

Short of restricting a cat or dog to an indoor existence, freedom from fleas is well nigh impossible.

Periodic spraying of an animal's intimate environment inside or outside the house may be helpful — especially if you are lucky and score a direct hit on a flea nest. However, keep in mind that flea eggs and pupae (the "adolescent" flea) are rather resistant to insecticides. It's the larvae, the "childhood" stage, that is the most vulnerable. For maximum effectiveness with the flea bomb it helps to have a degree in entomology. Of course, if you have an outdoor roamer then neither bomb nor degree will help much.

Flea collars? From the practical standpoint a joke. But serious business and ample earnings for the manufacturers. Millions are sold yearly. They don't really stop fleas. Or if they do, maybe only around the neck area where the collars may act as a local deterrent. There's still a lot of cat and dog left for the fleas to attack.

Collars contain insecticides which can and do cause chronic eye tearing and sneezing. When wet, these chemicals flush onto the skin and become absorbed into the body, posing a danger to a pet's nervous system. Some of the chemicals used in collars are spinoffs from nerve gas research.

Moreover, collars have been known to kill — not just fleas, but animals. In a 1975 study at Washington State University, five out of fifty cats eventually died who had become ill from the toxicity of flea collars. The surviving animals lost control of their bladders and rear legs, and became anemic and temperamental. Cats in particular have a lower tolerance than dogs to toxins of any kind.

Since those days the potency of collars has been modified. Nowadays they are hardly powerful enough to kill fleas. But in an allergy-prone animal the collar often causes a contact dermatitis — redness, itchiness, hair loss.

The latest gimmick is an ultra sound flea-killing device. Its safety and effectiveness have not yet been proven, however.

Many people feed their animals brewer's yeast in a misguided attempt to render animals flea-resistant. I haven't found it to work.

The yeast connection stems from the discovery that vitamin B-1 or brewer's yeast make humans "unpalatable" to insects. Yeast is a rich source of the B vitamins. Supposedly, when the B-1 component gets into your sweat glands it exudes a certain odor that turns off insects.

This trick may work for humans in the tropics or wherever insects abound but it doesn't help our pets. Dogs and cats have functional sweat glands between the toes. And that's it. If you want to keep fleas away from these peripheral parts then go ahead and feed yeast to your animal. But keep in mind that approximately 99 percent of the rest of the animal's body is open season for the flea.

Keep in mind also that yeast is not a wholly benign substance. In both humans and animals it is highly allergenic. I have treated many cats and dogs for allergic skin reactions after their owners fed them brewer's yeast. When the yeast was yanked, the skin usually improved.

If you regard the flea as a secondary problem, and treat the primaries, the flea becomes less of a menace. To be sure, trying to control and eliminate fleas in an animal's territory is important, but trying to make an animal less attractive to insects is a good idea as well.

Many times owners complain about flea infestations that defy all their best efforts to control. They bathe and spray their animals. They spray the carpets and the yard. Yet the fleas seem to thrive.

If an animal is unwell, no matter what the cause, insects seem to detect the weakness and go for that animal. I have found that if you correct diet and nutritional deficiencies, along with any immune system imbalances, you can create a virtual "flea proof" animal.

I have found mineral supplementation particularly effective. Fleas tend to shop elsewhere for blood when animals are on minerals. I have received many a call from penitent owners who said their animals became flea-ridden again after the minerals ran out and were not continued.

Food allergies and fleas often go together. I recall the case of a household of two Labs and one Golden Retriever. The latter dog was always having skin problems. One summer the animals were brought to my clinic. The Retriever's condition had become worse. He was full of fleas and pockets of red, raw itchy skin. The Labs seemed to have far fewer fleas and no reaction to speak of.

I started the Retriever on a hypoallergenic diet and the change was dramatic. Within a week the owner reported the scratching had lessened and the skin was beginning to heal. After two weeks, I re-examined the dog and his flea population was way down. His skin was indeed on the mend.

Here was a case of an animal apparently unable to tolerate a stressful diet. The reactions to food surfaced on the skin. He was a sick animal, a ripe target for fleas, who have the nose to find the least resistant animal in the household. The primary problem here was food allergies. The fleas were secondaries that merely aggravated the existing turmoil.

"Rusty," a five-year-old Irish setter, had been raised on high-protein kibble. The dog had chronically inflamed ears and feet, a rash on the stomach, and in the summer would develop a typical flea-allergy dermatitis over the base of the tail.

The dog was switched to a low-protein hypoallergenic diet. His skin quickly cleared up, despite the fact we made the change in the height of the flea season. There was still the occasional flea found on the dog but no more reaction. The priming food allergen was gone. The body could now tolerate a certain amount of the flea saliva allergen.

In many cases of flea-bite allergy there is a cortisol imbalance present. Such an animal has poor control of its immune cells. When the flea bite occurs, an overreaction takes place and shows up as irritated skin. When you correct the imbalance the overreaction stops, even if the fleas are still present. You have corrected the primary problem. The secondary has less impact. I have used this equation very successfully in treating many dogs and cats.

The standard treatment for flea-allergy dermatitis includes a steroid drug to reduce itching and inflammation. External lotions, sprays and powders are also used. When the medication is gone, signs of the flea-allergy often return. However, most veterinarians won't keep an animal indefinitely on steroids for fear of side-effects. But if the animal is cortisol deficient than the drug will produce few, if any, side-effects. Conversely, it should help keep the animal healthy and flea-resistant. In Chapter Seventeen I will provide the testing details to determine a cortisol deficiency along with suggestions on which types of steroids to use therapeutically.

EAR MITES

Ear mites are found throughout the animal kingdom. Rodents, dogs, wild and domesticated cats are all common carriers. The favorite food of these parasites is ear wax.

Mites are miniscule creatures and their presence is confirmed usually by microscopic identification.

The signs of an infestation are head shaking, ear scratching, and the appearance of a black, flecky-like bloody discharge in the ear canal. Often an owner will comment that an animal's ears are infected and bleeding.

A mite infestation can lead to localized infections with pockets of greenish-yellowish pus. This can spread to the inner ear and cause total deafness if not treated.

I have seen many households of multiple pets, particularly dogs, where one animal is affected and not the others. Just like the flea, mites have a knack for zeroing in on sick animals. I find that pets with food and skin-related allergies become prime targets since their conditions often impact in the ears. They will have red, inflamed ears and often a hypersecretion of wax. This is five-star dining for the mite.

Hunting dogs and outside cats, of course, can pick up a dose of mites as a natural consequence of roaming.

If you suspect ear mites, bring your animal to a veterinarian. This parasitic condition should be diagnosed professionally. Some people will rush out and buy an insecticide and do more damage than good to the animal. Insecticides can be irritating to a inflamed ear.

In my practice, I like to treat the inflammation and food allergy along with the mites. I get better results this way. I will put an animal on a hypoallergenic diet, check for trypsin deficiency, often supplement with trace minerals, and treat the ears topically.

MANGE

Called the red mange or generalized demodectic mange, this is another form of parasitic suffering generated by mites. Here the culprit is Demodex folliculorum, a mite who frequents hair follicles. He and his mates are permanent boarders, living deep among the follicles, where they thrive and propagate. Under the microscope, they resemble cigars with wheels.

Infestations usually starts on the head — typically around the eyes — or the extremities, and then spreads, sometimes affecting the whole trunk. Patchy hair loss, slight swelling and redness can develop into a bloody, miserable mess.

It is interesting to note that mites are present in probably 100 percent of the dog population. Normally, they live in peace with their surroundings, unseen and unheard from.

Eruption is believed to occur as a byproduct of an immune imbalance. One group of veterinary researchers found malfunctioning lymphocytes among animals with this problem. In their investigation the researchers took blood samples from affected animals. They separated the immune cells from bodily fluids and put them through a cleansing process. Following this laboratory "laundry," the lymphocytes appeared to regain their old fighting form again.

This experiment suggests to me there must be something in the blood causing the immune cell suppression. I wonder if that something might be an estrogen connection. In my research I have usually found a cortisol imbalance with high levels of adrenal estrogen in these animals. As I noted in Chapter Nine, too much estrogen can suppress the action of lymphocytes, the white blood cells that produce antibodies to combat disease.

The endocrine-immune imbalance may be an open invitation for mites. With a crippled immune system, any excess stress can quickly overload an animal's capacity to keep the parasites under control.

It is important to see a veterinarian as soon as possible. Infestations can spread rapidly. Delay can put an animal beyond the realm of help. Treatment involves the use of a powerful insecticide that can cause seizures. The greater the extent of the infestation the more of the chemical is needed. So don't wait for the condition to spread.

In treating mange I usually try to correct any hormonal imbalances and nutritional problems that may be involved.

INHALANT ALLERGIES

The typical signs of inhalant allergy are sneezing, runny eyes and nose, and sometimes scratching and rubbing of the head.

To test for specific allergens, veterinarians will often take an animal with an apparent inhalant problem and conduct an elaborate series of interdermal injections. This is similar to the "scratch tests" performed by allergy doctors. You put a bit of the substance under the skin and look for localized swelling. If a reaction occurs you have an indication of sensitivity to that substance. You send the findings to a laboratory which then develops an appropriate vaccine for the animal. Treatment usually includes injected or oral steroids along with topical preparations.

At one point I had developed a test that could monitor 175 different allergens, including human hair and dander, and seven Western and nine Southern grasses. I used this method extensively for years but was never really satisfied with it. I had mixed results.

My discovery of the endocrine-immune connection gave me a better tool with which to treat inhalant allergies.

I see quite a few referrals after skin testing and desensitization treatment have failed. Often the pet owner will tell me that "the dog seems better until we give him the shot and then he itches like hell for ten days afterward." Many times, people will stop the vaccine altogether because it seems to make the condition worse.

Why should it be? You have identified particular substances to which the immune system is sensitive. Then you inject them directly into the body expecting to switch on the production of appropriate antibodies.

The problem is this: many animals have the cortisol deficiency with an associated antibody imbalance. Their immune response is abnormal. They can't give you a textbook reaction to the injected allergen. The vaccination is like pouring gasoline on a fire.

But then again there are times the vaccination treatment will work. Or at least it seems to be working. In reality, it is the cortisone that is working and not the vaccinations. And for as long as you provide the cortisone accompaniment, the treatment seems to work. When you stop the cortisone you may simultaneously terminate the animal's ability to cope with the vaccination.

Cortisone fills a cortisol vacuum in an adrenal-defective animal. It permits a normal processing and buildup of antibodies to the vaccine. In these cases, the vaccine is secondary to the treatment just as the inhalant allergy is secondary to the existing imbalance.

In my clinic, I test first for the adrenal defect and correct that. This usually restores the animal's inherent ability to counteract the allergen without any vaccination at all.

When you treat the primary problem, the secondaries are much more manageable.

PART TWO

The Remedies

13

What — And What Not — To Do

On the following pages you will find a practical plan for enhancing health, accelerating the healing process, and preventing disease in your animals. On your own and with the good help of your veterinarian, there is a lot you can do about what ails your animals. But before you get started let me make a few important suggestions.

If an animal is experiencing major difficulty or suffering in an obvious way, be sure to get professional help first before you try anything on your own.

If your cat or dog is presently under the care of a veterinarian for a specific ailment then by all means continue that treatment. Do not stop. Consult with your veterinarian and discuss the ideas here as possible additions to ongoing therapy or alternatives to treatments that are maybe not yielding expected results.

If your animal has an allergic problem or two or is in generally acceptable health, then you can go ahead with Steps 1 and 2 on your own.

The first step is changing diet, providing your animal with the "cleanest" possible food. I will instruct you how to make simple hypoallergenic meals yourself or where to purchase ready-to-eat products that meet high standards.

The second step is extremely easy. You give your animal a readily obtainable mineral supplement that compensates for likely dietary deficiencies.

Step 3 requires a laboratory test for trypsin. It is advisable to have the test done just to make sure that what you feed your pet is being absorbed. Improper absorption is fairly common.

I recommend doing steps 1, 2 and 3 simultaneously. It's a shotgun approach but gets results faster. Once an animal is improved you may want to go back and play detective, that is, try the measures individually to see precisely which one is the most effective. It may be that your animal's health problem has more than just one cause. That's another reason for trying all three steps at once.

Step 4 is performed by a veterinarian and is intended primarily for chronically sick animals who do not respond to standard therapy or any of the measures I have just mentioned.

This step involves testing for cortisol, the vital adrenal hormone that is often deficient and usually overlooked in treatment programs. The deficiency renders animals highly vulnerable to allergies and serious diseases as well as interfering with the healing process. In Chapter Seventeen I have compiled detailed testing and evaluative information for veterinarians plus recommendations for safe and effective replacement therapy.

A large percentage of sick animals in my practice, otherwise unresponsive to treatment, have made excellent recoveries with hormonal replacements.

If your animal is basically healthy, you'll surely want to keep things that way. In the disease prevention chapter you will find practical suggestions for preserving optimal health. In that chapter I also want to share some concerns about cosmetic and fad breeding practices and how they adversely affect the health of purebreeds.

I feel disease prevention should begin with breeding programs.

The Plan — At a glance

Chapter Fourteen — Step 1 — The Hypoallergenic diet
Chapter Fifteen— Step 2 — Mineral supplementation
Chapter Sixteen— Step 3 — Enzyme supplementation
Chapter Seventeen — Step 4 — Hormonal Replacement
Chapter Eighteen — Disease prevention

14

The Hypoallergenic Diet

A hypoallergenic diet is a balanced food program that does not create adverse reactions in an animal. It generally excludes foods appearing on the Allergic HIT List in Chapter Three. The major offenders include beef, tuna, milk, eggs, brewers yeast, wheat, corn and chemical additives — items found in many commercial pet food formulations.

Over the last fifteen years I have developed a number of "clean" diets that provide unoffensive food while at the same time providing good nutrition. These diets have worked for many hundreds of cats and dogs I have treated in my clinic.

In one week you should be able to tell if the hypoallergenic diet is improving your animal's health. If chronic signs of allergy begin subsiding, that's a good indication you're on the right track. It tells you your animal was previously eating something that was causing problems.

One of the effective plans I use is the "Heidi Diet," a non-meat regimen. This diet was motivated by pure necessity rather than by any vegetarian philosophy. There are a number of animals who cannot remain for any length of time on meat of any sort — chicken, horsemeat, or even the least allergenic of meats, lamb. In my practice alone I have seen several hundred such pets. They may seem to do well on less allergenic meats for a while but eventually all the problems return. My first choice then for all allergic animals is the non-meat diet.

This may seem strange to you. Didn't dogs evolve primarily on a flesh diet? Partly true. They also ate many plant foods in the wilds.

Breeding practices of the recent past have caused many genetic changes in today's animals. They are no longer the stout-hearted creatures they once were. You can't put today's Labrador out in the field and expect him to be a natural hunter. Yesterday's meat-eater may be today's quiche-eater.

Keep in mind also that some animals may be intolerant to even the foods contained in my hypoallergenic programs. These dogs and cats are so genetically crippled they can hardly tolerate any food without experiencing an allergic reaction. In such cases, the information in Chapter Seventeen should be of great help.

Following are several diet plans. Take your pick.

DIETS FOR DOGS

1. Homemade recipes. Many small dogs in particular have very selective taste and will not eat commercial foods.

● Cottage cheese and rice. Many sensitive dogs seem to do OK on cottage cheese even though they are intolerant of dairy. Rice is perhaps the most digestible and least allergenic of grains and is an excellent source of carbohydrate (energy food). But whole grain brown rice, please. No denuded instant white rice. Prepare the rice as if you were eating it yourself. You can add a bit of garlic powder for flavor. If you have a small dog, cook enough rice at one time to last the entire seven day period. Store it in the refrigerator and warm up each day's portion. Add the cottage cheese. I recommend a half cup of cottage cheese to each cup or cup-and-a-half of rice. The portion would depend on the size of the animal. Feed twice a day.

● Lamb and rice. Among meats, I have found lamb is the least allergenic. You can use it in any form. I often recommend ground lamb. You make patties and braise them. Separately cook your brown rice. Then mix the two. Add garlic powder for flavor.

● "The Heidi Diet." I developed this dish years ago for "Heidi," the pet Doberman of Marcy and Bill Shatner. "Heidi" had a difficult time with meat. It caused debilitating gas that once temporarily paralyzed her rear legs. I have since recommended this recipe for many dogs who are intolerant to meat of any kind.

The recipe calls for two cups each of soy beans, brown rice, celery, and carrots, with one tablespoon of soy oil. Regular soy beans can be substituted with pre-cooked soy flakes for more convenience.

First you soak the soy beans overnight. In the morning you pour out the water and add fresh water, enough to more than cover the beans. Then boil until tender.

Meanwhile, cook the rice, using two cups of water for each cup of rice. Bring to a boil. Cover the rice and lower the flame. Cook on a low light until finished.

Mix the cooked rice and beans (or soy flakes) with the fresh vegetables. Add about a teaspoon of garlic powder for flavor. Bake it as a loaf for one hour at 350. Feed your animal twice a day according to the amount you would normally provide.

2. Prepared diets.

● Some years ago, I collaborated with a food manufacturer in order to have a good quality hypoallergenic diet readily available to pet owners. The result of this effort was a full line of both non-meat and meat preparations in can and dry form. I now use these products exclusively in my practice and obtain excellent dietary control with them.

You can ask your veterinarian or favorite pet or health food store to recommend a quality formulation for your hypoallergenic program. Try to purchase a product that does not contain any of the common allergens appearing on my HIT List. READ LABELS!

If you have a particularly finicky eater who balks at commercially prepared food, you might prepare a bit of lamb and add it to the store-bought formulation. A commercial baby food of lamb can also be used.

DIETS FOR CATS

When it comes to food, cats are persnickety creatures. So it's harder to design a restricted diet. You can create the best hypoallergenic diet in the world and your cat may not eat it.

1. Homemade recipes.
● Lamb and rice. Chicken and rice. Prepared the same as for dogs. The rice is optional. Often a cat will eat a raw and/or cooked ground lamb or chicken preparation.

If a cat is strictly fish-oriented and won't touch meat, you can trick him by mixing in some fish liver oil. I recommend a cold-pressed cod liver oil or a marine lipid oil readily available in health food stores. In my practice I prefer the marine lipid — from shark oil — since I have found some cats are sensitive to cod liver oil. I use one particular formula with good effect. You can find something similar at a health food store.

You can also use some garlic powder to create a seasoning that may appeal to the feline palate.

2. Prepared diets.
● I have been using the same brand of hypoallergenic foods I formulated years ago. You can find a good product for your animal by asking your veterinarian or neighborhood pet shop or health food store. You can enhance palatability with fish liver oil, garlic powder, or by adding some lamb or chicken.

● Use a baby food, either lamb or chicken based.

SIGNS OF IMPROVEMENT

Seven days is enough time on a hypoallergenic diet to see many chronic problems getting better. Look for improvement in these areas:
● itchy, scratchy skin.
● biting and chewing of skin.
● inflamed ears.

- diarrhea and loose stool.
- vomiting.

Be alert. Watch for less itching and scratching, for more solid stools. Look for improvement of any of the chronic difficulties affecting your animal.

An animal with skin problems may develop dandruff after starting this program. That's a good sign. The flakiness often accompanies a healing skin. If improvement is in progress, there is also less scratching.

WHAT TO DO NEXT

If you see your animal getting better, continue the diet for another seven days.

At that point you can continue indefinitely on the hypoallergenic diet or, as I often recommend, use this diet as a base and carefully test other foods that can be added to it. I call this phase the "add-back plan."

It works like this:

Select a food, preferably one not on the Hit List, and add it alone to the hypoallergenic base diet for a week. If there are no signs of returning allergy you can assume that the particular food is tolerated.

I suggest starting with a homemade food first, perhaps chicken the first week. Prepared it at home. If there are no reactions find a commercial chicken product for pets and test it the same way the following week. Make sure the contents include no common allergenic items. Read the ingredient label. Look out for chemical additives. See if the animal does as well as on the homemade chicken. I have known many pets who flourished on home cooking but did poorly on the commercial stuff.

You can continue to add back any food to your animal's diet once the food has passed the seven day test. You can then rotate, mix and ad lib within the boundaries of tolerated foods.

But remember — add back only one food per week.

If you want more ideas on creating healthy homemade concoctions for your animals, get a copy of a delightful book by food expert-author Frances Sheridan Goulart: "Bone Appetite! Natural Foods for Pets." The book, replete with tasty and imaginative recipes, is available (at $2.95) at many health food stores or through the publisher — Pacific Search Books, 715 Harrison Street, Seattle, WA 98109. Some of the recipes, however, have allergenic foods. Watch for the no-no's and treat them with caution.

ADDED ADVICE

- If your animal is on any program of medication, don't stop it.
- Eliminate any chew sticks, vitamins, biscuits, or snacks. Any one of these items can be the cause of allergic reactions. In the hypoallergenic diet program, all foods and nutritional supplements are guilty until proven innocent.
- Don't cheat! Be honest. You may not think so, but even a small

amount of a treat can be devastating.

● Try to keep your animal away from other food during the test. Be aware of well-meaning friends and relatives who might toss a piece of meat or chocolate in your animal's direction.

● Table scraps are OK as long as they are foods you know are tolerated by your animal. Mix them into the regular food.

● Be careful of overloading your animal's digestive tract. I recommend feeding two or three times daily rather than heaping one large meal into the dinner bowl. This will serve a couple of important purposes.

For one, it will keep the animal satisfied throughout the day so he won't be strongly motivated to seek food elsewhere.

Secondly, the single-meal overload has a sludging effect and can overwhelm an animal's biochemical and mechanical ability to process food — even if the meal is hypoallergenic. Overloading by itself can create signs of allergy such as loose stool, vomiting and skin problems.

15

Mineral Supplementation

Mineral deficiencies — severe or just even subtle — are often involved in health problems. That's why I recommend my clients give their animals a good natural supplement. I believe minerals are so important that I suggest supplementation whether an animal is sick or not.

If you are starting your pet on the hypoallergenic diet, go right ahead and begin the mineral supplement as well. It can bring improvement faster.

I use a formula made from a natural occuring precipitate obtained from ancient sea beds in Nevada. It contains 72 different minerals. Included are familiar names such as calcium, magnesium, manganese, potassium, iron and zinc, and some not-so-familiar names like wolfram, niobium, scandium, lanthanum, and gadolinium.

The mineral precipitate developed over eons from countless levels of crustacean life forms deposited one atop the other. Over time, rains leached this ancient graveyard and created a uniformity of micron-sized crystals, loosely bonded with electrically-charged minerals.

Due to the physical structure of this compound, mineral particles are easily dissolved and readily pass through the intestinal barrier into the bloodstream. Thus, the minerals in the compound are chelated by nature — that is, bound to organic substances for pickup and use by the body as needed.

The chelation factor makes this compound most attractive for replacement therapy and general dietary supplementation. There need be no concern for dogs on low sodium diets and cats on low ash diets. Their intestines will uptake and utilize only what the body needs. The remainder of the minerals will pass out in the feces.

In Chapter Six I described the many benefits I see in animals who are supplemented with this type of formula.

HOW TO ADMINISTER

There are many naturally chelated multi-mineral compounds available through health food stores or veterinarians.

Mineral formulas come in either powder or tablet form. Read the label for proper dosages. This is determined usually by weight of the animal.

Powder can be mixed right into the food and that's probably the easiest and most efficient way to administer the minerals. If an animal is ultra fussy, just start with a lower dose and work up slowly to the recommended level.

Some cats don't like the gritty texture that powder adds to food. In that case you can try pilling. Your veterinarian can tell you how to do it. If, however, you or your animal are not comfortable with pilling, don't do it.

If pilling isn't practical, then simply drop tablets in the animal's water where they will dissolve.

Supplements should be taken on a daily basis.

16

Topping Up The Enzymes

Even a good hypoallergenic diet along with trace mineral supplementation may not solve nutritional and digestive causes of disease if an absorption problem is present.

Trypsin, as I explained in Chapter Seven, is an unheralded enzyme produced by the pancreas that plays a large role in the digestive breakdown of carbohydrates, fats and also protein. Many animals have major or minor trypsin deficiencies which tie up traffic in the gut and prevent proper absorption of nutrients.

The classic signs of a complete deficiency are significant weight loss despite a larger than normal appetite and passing much more stool than normal.

More often than not, fractional shortages are involved. Something less than an ideal amount is supplied by the pancreas. Just a small deficiency is enough to create allergic problems.

Combined with the hypoallergenic diet and trace mineral supplementation, I highly recommend that you have your animal tested for trypsin. It's a simple matter.

I think it's a good idea even if you have a healthy animal. If the deficiency is subtle, you are possibly not going to see the clinical signs for two or three years. So why not head off the headaches. As part of your animal's yearly checkup, include a trypsin test. The cost is minor.

All you need for the test is to provide your veterinarian with a sample of the animal's stool. The fecal test is used widely in veterinary practices. Recently, a blood test has been developed. It gives a more accurate reading but at this time it is also more expensive to perform.

After testing the stool, the veterinarian will indicate the degree, if any, of deficiency. Depending on the findings, an ennzyme supplement may be recommended.

The supplement is available either in tablet or powder form.

Many of the enzyme supplements that are sold are derived from dessicated pork pancreas. If your animal is allergic to pork you should stay away from such sources — otherwise you may be inviting problems or using a supplement that will have no effect whatsoever.

I use a product in my practice containing protease, amylase, and lipase, the other major pancreatic enzymes, which replace and compensate for the insufficient trypsin.

Signs of improvement often come fast. Usually the first indicator is a reduced amount of stool or perhaps harder-appearing stool. You may notice this within a week.

If there has been a weight loss problem, you can weigh the animal over a several week period and determine any weight gain as a result of the supplementation. This is a sign of improved digestion and utilization of foodstuffs.

The last sign of improvement to appear would be healthier skin and hair coat.

17

Hormone Replacement Therapy

This chapter is essentially for the veterinarian. It contains technical information on testing for and treating the endocrine-immune imbalance that is destroying the health of large segment of our pet population.

The guidelines for treatment are relatively uniform once a blood test has revealed the irregularities.

The procedure described here was first developed almost fifteen years ago and evolved to its present form over some 8,000 cases.

I strongly recommend applying this modality to all chronically allergic and ill animals and especially to stubborn cases unresponsive to standard treatment.

For cats, I find hormonal replacement particularly useful for FeLV, FIP, FUS, generalized and food allergies, dermatitis (including milliary dermatitis, flea allergy dermatitis, feline acne, neuromas, and eosinophilic granulomatous disease), and gingival disease leading to early loss of teeth.

For dogs: generalized allergy, dermatitises, generalized demodectic mange, chronic diseases of the liver, kidney, and pancreas, epilepsy, diseases of reproduction (false pregnancies-cystic ovaries, sterility, silent heats, abortions), chronic weight loss, chronic gastroenteritis and food allergies, and gingival diseases.

Concurrently with this replacement therapy, I recommend maintaining an animal on a hypoallergenic diet (Chapter Fourteen), along with trace mineral supplementation (Chapter Fifteen) and, if necessary, enzyme supplementation (Chapter Sixteen) to ensure good absorption of food and medication.

Turmoil in the gut, caused by food allergens or deficiencies of minerals or enzymes, can create a malabsorption situation. To obtain proper hormonal blood levels under such conditions you might be administering too much medication. The consequences could well be undesirable side effects and an improperly regulated animal. I get maximum results when I first clear up these details before attempting to replace hormones.

It is important to test for and correct the endocrine-immune imbalance as early as possible to prevent serious damage to organs by aggressive disease processes, such as feline leukemia and infectious peritonitis. Delay can reduce the effectiveness of this therapeutic approach.

HOW TO TEST

The testing method involves a simple blood test.

Two blood samples are taken — the first between 8 and 11 a.m., the second two hours later. After the second draw, the animal can be picked up and returned home.

The first sample represents a baseline biochemical profile before the activities and stresses of the day can affect and alter key measurements. There is no need for fasting. Animals should be treated normally before they are brought for testing. If normal routine includes an a.m. feeding then this should be provided at home as usual.

Immediately after the first blood draw the animal is given an IM injection of pituitary ACTH. Do not feed the animal between blood draws.

The ACTH stimulates the middle layer of the adrenal cortex to secrete cortisol. After two hours, when the second blood draw is taken, this stimulation effect is completed and the released cortisol is present in the peripheral blood supply.

The blood draw schedule at a glance:
- First draw, 8 to 11 a.m.
- Follow immediately with ACTH injection.
- Second draw, two hours later.

Instruct the laboratory to provide the following from the first draw:
- Complete blood count.
- Resting plasma cortisol. (Not a serum cortisol reading because you may obtain non-specific protein binding which can falsify the cortisol level).
- Estrogen
- T-3
- T-4
- IgA
- IgM
- IgG

and the following from the second blood draw:
- The ACTH-stimulated plasma cortisol.

Do not perform this test on a female in estrus so as to avoid the possibility of ovarian-source estrogen distorting the reading.

HOW TO READ TEST RESULTS

The most constant finding is the imbalance in cortisol, the result of a genetic adrenal defect. It is basically from this starting point that related biochemistry turns sour.

The values I regard as normal are probably going to differ from textbook standards you may be more familiar with. The reason is that standard norms are taken as isolated averages. I base my norms on comparisons to estrogen and

Endocrine-Immune Values

Cats — normal ranges		Dogs — normal ranges
l.0-2.5 ug/dl	*Rest cortisol*	l.0-2.5 ug/dl
15-24 ug/dl	*ACTH cortisol*	15-24 ug/dl
	●	
	Total estrogen	
20-25 pg/ml	-males-	20-25 pg/ml
30-35 pg/ml	-females-	30-35 pg/ml
	(ovario-hysterectomized or anestrus)	
	●	
37-50%	*T-3*	37-54%
1.5-5.4 ug %	*T-4*	1.7-4.0 ug %
70-160 mg/dl	*IgA*	70-160 mg/dl
100-200 mg/dl	*IgM*	100-200 mg/dl
1000-2000 mg/dl	*IgG*	1000-2000 mg/dl

antibody levels and how they are influenced by both active and inactive (bound) cortisol. Relationships, rather than simple individual values, are important to the interpretation of this test and to the subsequent success of the therapy.

● Cortisol Interpretation

It is very important to suspect that normal-appearing or high levels of cortisol may actually be inactive or bound cortisol and totally unusable to the body.

Very high levels of resting cortisol (over l0) with an ensuing surge (to over 25 and 30) in the ACTH-stimulated level would probably be considered a case of Cushing's Syndrome.

However, Cushing's may not be involved at all.

The presence of lymphocytes and eosinophils in the CBC is a biochemical clue that cortisol may be inactive. Further proof would be high levels of adrenal estrogen and antibodies.

From all appearances you think you are seeing Cushing's, but the real story is an insidious, inactive hormone that serves little use but does considerable harm.

In this situation, administration of Lysodren (OPDDD), the standard treatment for Cushing's, would severely hurt an animal. Lysodren destroys adrenal cortical tissue. This is how you bring cortisol levels down to a more normal range. You can imagine then the adverse effect — death, perhaps — resulting from further suppression of already defective adrenal tissue.

Over the years I have found very high levels of bound cortisol in about a dozen dogs and then successfully treated them with cortisone. If the cortisol was not bound, cortisone would obviously be contra-indicated.

The CBC is necessary to supply a comprehensive picture. It indicates whether you have a bound, inactive cortisol or not. If you test for cortisol alone you are likely to miss important clues. You see just a fragment of the truth.

I like to see a resting cortisol level between 1.0 and 2.5. However, there are factors which can alter these values: an animal who is stressed or is currently on cortisone medication.

● Estrogen Interpretation

Estrogen can exert a dramatic blocking effect on cortisol and thyroid hormones.

Too much estrogen production transforms fully potent cortisol into an inactive form called transcortin.

Similarly, too much or too little estrogen deactivates thyroid secretions. The blood levels of T-3 and T-4 may show as perfectly normal yet the hormones can be rendered useless because of estrogen irregularities. This phenomenon has been misleading for years to veterinarians.

Estrogen just a point or two out of the normal range is enough to cause varying degrees of these complications.

● T-3 and T-4 Interpretation

Deviations of these compounds suggest a hypo or hyper condition relating to the genetic makeup of the individual dog or cat.

Levels can appear totally normal yet be largely unusable to the body if estrogen is too high or low. You must then prescribe an outside source of thyroid for the animal, enough to overcome the estrogenic block.

Be alert to the possibility of a secondary anemia. This might occur from estrogen levels that are too high.

● Antibody Interpretation

IgA is the mucous membrane antibody. An abnormally high or low level is often involved in food allergies and malabsorption. This imbalance can also interfere with intestinal absorption of orally-administered medication and replacement hormones. I will talk more about this problem later on in my treatment discussion.

IgM is the first line of antibody defense, acting as a roadblock against incoming micro-organisms and other foreign invaders until more specialized antibodies can be produced.

IgM is regulated in part by cortisol. With a cortisol deficiency, this antibody level is often too high. When estrogen is too high, IgM may become suppressed. When such hormonal situations are normalized, the IgM level returns to normal.

Too much or too little IgM saps resistance to disease.

IgG is the specific antibody produced by lymphocytes against specific agents in the body. IgG reacts abnormally to irregularities of cortisol and estrogen and therefore provides another measurement of lymphocyte behavior. Levels too high or too low, just as with IgA and IgM, invite disease.

RECOMMENDATIONS FOR MEDICATION

I have found that medication-by-weight ratios are often invalid because of individual differences. One animal may respond to one unit of a given preparation and the next may require ten.

I believe in titrating conservatively. The key to success is to prescribe just enough to create homeostasis. You also lessen the possibility of side effects. Keep in mind you are likely providing hormones for a lifetime, not just treating short-term for elimination of clinical signs. Temporarily, you can use powerful levels of medication but for the long run, for perhaps 10 or 15 years, you want dosages as optimal and safe as possible.

● Replacement Preparations

1. Cortisol. Prednisolone is my first choice for cortisol replacement. Often by itself it solves many problems. It is usually administered once a day. The lowest possible levels are used to promote normalization, starting as low as 1 mg to 5 mg. Dosage is increased according to need and safety.

If the cat or dog has any side effects, such as excess thirst, urination or appetite, incontinence, a general apathy or lethargy, or panting at night, I then recommend using Medrol. I start with 1 mg and titrate up to an effective level, which can be verified by retesting the estrogen and antibody levels after some two months on the program. Medrol is not as potent or effective as Prednisolone. However, it usually does not produce side effects.

I estimate about 30 percent of dogs and 10 percent of cats will require Medrol. The majority do well with Prednisolone.

2. Thyroid. If thyroid is deficient or estrogen levels abnormally high or low, then thyroid replacement is necessary in conjection with Prednisolone (or Medrol).

Synthroid (Flint) is the only preparation I use. The generic — l-thyroxine — is not as effective.

My general recommendation is to begin with approximately .1 mg per 20 pounds of body weight, half the suggested dosage.

For dogs I prescribe this amount twice a day, morning and evening.

For cats with high or low estrogen levels, once a day is adequate. However, if thyroid levels are low I prescribe Synthroid twice daily.

I found that many animals respond nicely to conservative dosage. Additionally there is less chance of side effects.

Dosage can be slowly increased until desired results are obtained.

Of all my cases, I found that less than 1 percent could not tolerate Synthroid. If dosage is too high, or the animal is simply intolerant, the signs are these: hyperexcitability, irritability, elevated heart rate and fever, vomiting and diarrhea. There are other types of thyroid preparation available in case Synthroid is not appropriate.

3. Estrogen. A subnormal level means that the inner layer of the adrenal cortex is genetically damaged.

Once you start cortisol replacement, the estrogen level will decrease even more. That's because ACTH activity is restored to normal by the cortisone. There is then less stimulation of the inner layer cortex by the ACTH and therefore less estrogen being squeezed out.

This situation generally requires estrogen replacement only in a spayed female where cortisol replacement has led to incontinence. Estrogen should be raised to a normal level or to the level of continence. This can be done by using 1 mg tablets of estrogen. I use 1 tablet daily in the morning for 5 days. If the dribbling and incontinence stops, then I go to 1 tablet every other day for 3 periods. I continue in that mode so as to use as little estrogen as necessary. In a majority of cases the animals get along nicely on 1 tablet twice a week.

Remember — if estrogen therapy is excessive, you will recreate the original cortisol imbalance.

REPLACEMENT THERAPY — CATS

Cats will usually require more medication per body weight than dogs to regulate their mechanism.

● FeLV

While attempting to treat this condition and change the underlying adrenal mechanism, the cat should be receiving fluids and whatever support therapy is indicated.

I begin with a minimum of 10 mg Prednisolone daily. If there is no response within 2 days I go to 20 mg. If there is no response after 2 more days I then add .1 mg of Synthroid once a day.

Should these measures still not bring a positive response after two more days, I resort to injectable Prednisolone and continue the Synthroid as before. If the cat has a known absorption problem, I bypass oral cortisone altogether. Dose levels are the same.

A high or low IgA reading on the blood test indicates an absorption problem. If this is the case, begin with an injectable.

If the blood test reveals a low thyroid hormone level, then start immediately with the Synthroid — .1 mg morning and evening.

When signs of recovery are seen it is crucial to continue the replacement therapy. The defect you are addressing is a permanent one and the disease is an endproduct of that condition. Do not back off once the cat starts to improve. If you cut back on the cortisone while the the virus is still present in the body you are essentially disarming the cat. The imbalance will recur and permit the disease to resume its destructive path. You probably have to replace the missing cortisol for the rest of the animal's life.

Many cats will shed the virus totally or to a large degree as they regain full health. They will test negative for the virus, contrary to popular belief.

I have seen cats shed the virus and test negative after six weeks. With some it has taken two years. And still with others, there is always a pesky residual virus present — but no signs. I have been able to control about 80 percent of several hundred symptomatic FeLV cases by correcting the hormonal mechanisms.

Once the cat is flourishing you will want to check the antibody and estrogen levels. At about four to six weeks, do another blood test. If the levels are still high then the cat requires more cortisol replacement. If too low, that means too much cortisone is being supplied and you will want to cut back. By bringing these biochemical markers into the normal range you can individualize and fine focus the replacement process. This is your insurance against the side effects of long-term steroid therapy. You can monitor the biochemical situation with follow-up blood tests at six month or yearly intervals.

I should mention here the possibility — I have seen it only rarely — of adrenal cortex resurrection and the resumption of normal cortisol production again. A drop in the estrogen and antibody levels in follow-up testing would give you the clue. You would then back off on the cortisone. A continuing normalization of the estrogen and antibody levels tells you that indeed the adrenal cortical layer is functioning again.

● FIP

I have found FIP more resistant to therapy than FeLV. Nevertheless, the replacement program has achieved good control in about 70 percent of cases thus far.

Treatment is basically the same as in feline leukemia with a couple of important differences.

I find many FIP cats have trypsin deficiencies and an absorption problem. Because of this, oral medication often works poorly or not at all. Thus it is advisable to use injectable Prednisolone in the early stages.

This may help explain why FIP is more resistant and especially why supplying proper food, enzymes and trace minerals is essential. I will routinely add enzymes to the cat's food whether I identify a deficiency or not. I believe this makes a big difference.

Once a cat shows signs of recovery, oral medication can be cautiously substituted.

Any abnormal fluid concentration in the lungs or abdomen that is causing clinical difficulty should be drained off. Clinical signs would dictate any other intervention.

● FUS

IgA, the antibody active in mucous membranes throughout the body, including the bladder and urethra lining, may turn up in the blood test as abnormally high or low values when FUS is involved. IgM and IgG may also be abnormal.

The IgA situation underscores the importance of a hypoallergenic diet. Food allergens can stimulate an irregular IgA reaction, and, in the case of the urinary tract, contribute to chronic irritation and stone formation.

Follow the replacement routine as described for FeLV. Provide any medication which may be necessary.

● Skin problems and allergies (generalized dermatitis, flea-allergy dermatitis, feline acne, neuromas, eosinophilic granulomas, milliary dermatitis).

Again, follow the FeLV regimen. These conditions respond nicely to therapy. Once you recreate endocrine-immune homeostatis, disease signs generally subside. But you must continue the replacement therapy and that can be for the entire life of the cat.

The majority of the skin problems are directly associated with a cortisol deficiency and a hyperimmunity — lost control of the immune cells. The antibodies, as seen in the tests, all tend to be elevated. Sometimes there are combinations where two out of the three will be high but for the most part they are all abnormally high.

Replacement usually involves Prednisolone by itself. Occasionally, there may be an estrogen involvement.

● Other chronic diseases unresponsive to standard therapy (including gingival disease).

Follow the FeLV example.

REPLACEMENT THERAPY — DOGS

● Chronic allergic dermatitises (including flea-allergy dermatitis).

These conditions are variably characterized by endless scratching, gnawing, biting, and chewing of skin, by redness, thickness, flakiness, itchiness, coarseness, and by hair loss.

Cortisol deficiency is usually involved. Dogs are hyperimmune. Their antibodies exceptionally high. Sometimes these factors are combined with elevated or depressed estrogen, or thyroid deficiency.

In dogs less than 10 pounds, start with a dose of 1 mg to 2.5 mg Prednisolone orally once a day. Increase 1 mg each following day.

If side effects occur within a day or two, Prednisolone should be substituted with Medrol. The Medrol starting dose is 1 mg daily. Since Medrol may not be as effective, you may want to increase it every day or two by .5 or 1 mg to reach desired effect. Medrol is administered in the morning.

In dogs over 10 pounds, begin with 2.5 mg Prednisolone. Usually between 2.5 and 10 mg a day is adequate unless antibody levels are exceptionally high — as they frequently are. In this case, it takes longer to reduce the hyperreactivity of the lymphocytes.

If you reach 10 mg a day and the dog is still having problems, you can increase the dose to 15 mg every other day. One day you give 10, the next day 15, etc. I have found this to be a a safe and effective way of gaining control over a stubborn situation. You can even safely kick up the alternate days to 20 mg or more. Then, as you are begin to see improvement, you back off the increased alternate day dose. You can shave the high doses by stepping down to, say, 17.5, then 15, then 12.5, and then remaining constantly at 10 or whatever level is effective in the particular case. If clinical signs have subsided and remain under control, you have properly regulated the lymphocytes.

If 2 or 3 weeks go by without noticeable control, recheck the antibodies with another blood test. If antibody levels have not gone down there may be an absorption problem. Medication is not getting through.

To get around an intestinal roadblock use injections or an absorption-enhancing procedure I will describe immediately following the dog section.

As with cats, a too high or too low estrogen level will effect thyroid hormone function, even if the latter levels appear normal. For dogs, the combination of Prednisolone with Synthroid is highly effective. In such a situation, Prednisolone by itself without a thyroid replacement is much less effective.

Most veterinarians know that after you start an animal on Prednisolone the medication will work fine for a given period of time. Then, more and more is needed to obtain the same results. Eventually, it doesn't work at all. The thinking has been that the body becomes resistant to the medication.

I'm not so sure about that. I believe Prednisolone acts sluggishly because of the thyroid block caused by estrogen. Introduction of Synthroid — substituting for the inactivated thyroid hormone — elevates metabolism and permits Prednisolone to act more effectively to regulate lymphocyte activity. The influence of the estrogen is overcome.

I recommend half of the normally-suggested dosage of Synthroid. I begin with .1 mg per 20 pounds of body weight, given orally twice a day, a.m. and p.m. After two weeks, raise the amount to .15 mg twice a day...and so on to reach desired effect.

In a spayed female, I sometimes need to use estrogen replacement as well as Prednisolone and Synthroid. A low estrogen level will drop even further once replacement therapy has begun. This is due to the ACTH-cortisol feedback. Without adequate cortisol, excess ACTH overstimulates adrenal estrogen. After replacement, the ACTH output normalizes, resulting in less estrogen secretion. This can lead to incontinence in a spayed female. If this occurs, the animal should receive estrogen.

Begin with 1 mg in the morning for 5 days. If the incontinence is corrected, drop to 1 mg every other day for 3 periods. Then decrease to 1 mg every third day, etc., in a continuing attempt to find the minimum effective level of estrogen. Most dogs will take 1 or 2 tablets weekly to correct this problem.

In large dogs 2 mg or more are sometimes necessary. Increase as needed.

Be conservative, however, because if you overdose with estrogen you can recreate the original biochemical imbalance. If, after estrogen is introduced and clinical signs of the original disease return, it is advisable to retest the animal in order to help determine a more effective estrogen level.

● Generalized demodectic mange

I find a definite cortisol connection in this disease complexity.

In many quarters, the use of steroids for mange is regarded as sinful. Here is an immune deficiency condition and by administering steroids, so the thinking goes, you suppress the immune system even more.

My investigations reveal that the majority of afflicted dogs are cortisol deficient. There is often a high level of estrogen as well, which can be very damaging. There is in fact an elevated antibody level, not a decreased level.

Associated with the disease is a transitory suppression of the thymic lymphocytes (T-cells). In laboratory studies, T-cells have been removed from canine serum and put through a "washing" process. In vitro, the "clean" T-cells have been found to have restored function. Something therefore in the blood is crippling these immune cells. I suggest an excessively high level of estrogen may be the villain.

My suggested treatment program:

1. Correct the hormonal imbalances. Use only enough Prednisolone to return the mechanism to normal. Often Synthroid is also indicated. Follow the therapy example for canine skin conditions.

2. Provide a good shampoo — such as Mitoban — to reduce the mange population.

3. Start a hypoallergenic diet.

4. Check for an enzyme problem.

5. Supplement with trace minerals.

6. Spay the female.

● Reproductive disorders (females) — false pregnancies-cystic ovaries, sterility, silent heats, abortions.

This can be a very defiant array of hormonally-linked problems often imitating allergies, often unresponsive to standard treatments, and often manifesting in subtle, misleading signs.

One of the most confusing sequences begins with a mild swelling and enlargement of the mammary glands occurring about a month after the end of the heat cycle. Frequently accompanying this is a hair loss, non-specific itching and scratching, and a loss of appetite. There is sometimes a behavioral change in which the animal will "adopt" a toy or person and begin digging and nesting as if she is about to whelp. Mammary tumors and pyometra may develop.

This condition presents various faces: an animal can pass through silent heats where there are no external signs of estrus, or become sterile, or become pregnant and after two or three weeks abort, or become a "nymphomaniac" and begin mounting other dogs.

In the best interest of the animal's health and to interrupt the aberrant hormonal cycle, it is advisable first to do a complete ovario-hysterectomy. This measure also prevents a genetic predisposition being passed on to offspring.

Spaying will clear up a number of these associated problems. If, after several weeks, there is a continuation of signs then the adrenal hormone complex needs to be tested and corrected. This would indicate that the ovaries were not primary agents in the problem, but secondary to the adrenal imbalance.

If the ovaries are not taken out first, the hormones they produce often tend to neutralize the replacement therapy.

If it is essential to breed the dog, first test for the hormonal mechanism. Try to determine where the problem is. Then correct it with proper replacement therapy.

It is important to find a male who does not have a tendency to throw female puppies with histories of sterility or cystic ovaries. Once the male is selected, perform the adrenal mechanism test on that animal as well. If the male has the adrenal imbalance, I strongly advise against mating the two animals. A union of two such adrenally-crippled dogs will perpetuate the problem and guarantee early disease in the offspring. Using this approach offers a method for identifying the problem and breeding it out. I frankly feel that any animal with the adrenal defect should not be bred so as to stop proliferation of the problem.

Most of these females are cortisol deficient. There is usually an inner layer cortical defect as well — meaning an associated estrogen imbalance. This leads to many sterility and reproductive problems. Antibody levels are typically high.

The widespread belief is that an animal will abort if you administer cortisone to the problem female during estrus, breeding and pregnancy. In reality, the animal may actually require regulatory cortisone. That is the case if the blood test shows a low cortisol level. Sterility and miscarriage are promoted if the animal has normal cortisol and you then administer cortisone.

● Idiopathic epilepsy.

I have found that many cases of epilepsy[7] seem to be triggered by foods — high protein diets, allergenic foods, changes in diet.

The blood test typically shows an animal deficient in cortisol and high or low in estrogen. Additionally, there are imbalances in the antibody levels and specifically in the food-related antibody, IgA, which can be either high or low. This mechanism is what creates the hypersensitivity to food and, I suggest, the biochemistry conducive for seizures.

An animal with this problem needs to be hormonally corrected and placed on a hypoallergenic diet.

I can often control seizures through hormonal replacement and diet without the use of anti-epileptic medication. If medication is required, it is considerably more effective if the hormonal imbalances are rectified and a non-provocative diet initiated.

● Chronic diseases unresponsive to standard therapy.

Test for the imbalances and treat according to the formula suggested above for skin problems.

WHAT TO DO IF IT DOESN'T WORK

Over the years I have had my share of hard nuts that wouldn't crack. With the exception of FeLV and FIP cases, I found that about 5 percent of the animals I treated with replacement therapy were not responding as expected. For FeLV and FIP, the percentage is higher.

One day about ten years ago I sat down with a stack of records —cases of unresponsive cats and dogs. I found I had duly followed the clues offered by the blood test and made the indicated hormonal replacements. I had prescribed good diet, trace minerals, enzymes, and whatever medication was necessary. But the results were poor. Retesting showed insignificant or no change in biochemical markers.

Going over this file of frustration I discovered a common denominator: IgA imbalances. That suggested poor absorption and interference with uptake of food, supplements and medication.

"Teal," the family Doberman, was in this category. She had skin problems and was down to thirty-five pounds. I was desperately trying to find a solution to save her from wasting away or having to put her to sleep.

I decided to try a combination of Azulfidine and pancreatic enzymes. The former is a drug for people with ulcerative colitis which I felt might normalize the mucous membrane lining of the gut. I hoped the enzymes would enhance enzymatic processing of food and replacement hormones.

Happily for "Teal" and the family, I got lucky on the first try. The IgA levels quickly started to normalize. With continued care and treatment I was able to save our Dobie and have since used this approach with good success on other recalcitrant cases.

I use one-half tablet of Azulfidine for twenty pounds of body weight, twice daily, mixed into the animal's food or directly pilled when other medication is administered.

As for the enzymes, simply follow the dosage directions on the label of the product you use.

Hormones are replaced as appropriate.

Usually you will see improvement of clinical signs within seven days.

In some cases you can avoid dealing with the gut altogether and go directly to injections. However, this is not a practical long-term solution for two reasons:

1. I have not found a form of Synthroid that is injectable.

2. The gut has to be normalized in any case otherwise the animal cannot utilize food well.

There is an important lesson for us to "absorb" here. Unsuccessful treatment of animals may not be a case of wrong or ineffective medication. Rather it may reflect an intestinal blockade — an inability for medicine to bridge the barrier between gut and bloodstream. An animal can't stay well if it can't absorb its medication.

In those hard nut cases, I will usually suspect a malabsorption problem or a non-compliant owner.

When a therapy program doesn't work, I will retrace my steps to see if I have made a mistake. If there is no mistake, I will question the owner to make sure the routine is being carefully followed. I check to see if the pharmacist may have given the less effective l-Thyroxine instead of Synthroid.

Often an owner forgets or is less diligent or is cheating on the program. Sometimes the dog or cat is getting into another animal's food, eating something of an allergenic nature. Or somebody in the house is feeding forbidden food. Such lapses are enough to upset the therapy.

This program has to be done 100 percent. I usually ask for a total commitment. If I can't get it, I don't start it.

Sometimes I will encounter pathetic animals so genetically damaged or so systemically diseased that nothing works for them.

WHAT ABOUT LONG-TERM STEROIDS?

"Patches" was a two-year-old Siamese. She had been diagnosed for FeLV by another veterinarian and given a few months to live. She had enlarged lymph nodes, hair loss, dermatitis, was not eating and had lost a large amount of weight. The cat had a history of flea allergies and generalized skin problems.

I took blood, checked for imbalances, and found a cortisol irregularity. This situation had left "Patches" vulnerable to the leukemia virus.

I started her on 20 mg of Prednisolone. The response was dramatic. It was as if a new cat was created. Her weight increased. Hair began to return. The lymph nodes regressed in size. The cat started talking amd becoming more social.

I now prescribed a lower dosage of Prednisolone to maintain homeostasis. I told the owner to keep "Patches" on this program indefinitely.

In time the cat regained full health.

Here was a happily-ever-after story until one day a friend of the owner told her that prolonged steroids was dangerous. So the owner stopped the program.

With the support system removed, the cat was left vulnerable once again with its defective adrenal mechanism. Before long, the old problems returned, including the virus.

The owner brought the sick cat back. "They told me steroids would kill the cat so I stopped the medication," she said.

I explained to her why this isn't so. "For sure your cat will die if you don't keep her on steroids," I said.

The owner resumed the therapy, first with 20 mg, and then maintenance on 10. The cat is now twelve-years-old, still on Pred, and has been healthy throughout the years.

Another time I was visited by the owner of a champion Bulldog. The animal had a history of false pregnancies and miscarriages. One time only did she produce a puppy and it was a genetic monstrosity.

I checked the bitch and found a cortisol deficiency. I started her on Prednisolone and Synthroid with appropriate diet and other supportive therapy.

The dog was maintained on this program. The owner eventually bred the female to a male who had a clean hormonal profile. The result was a litter of eight puppies, all healthy, and some of them now champions.

Word spread. Another Bulldog owner called me. He had a bitch with similar problems. I tested the dog and found the same imbalances. Replacement therapy was initiated.

The bitch was bred and became duly pregnant. X-ray examination was made at six-and-a-half weeks and revealed she was carrying five puppies. Two weeks later, I checked again to see if a Caesarean Section would be necessary. To my shock, there were no puppies. They had aborted.

I questioned the owner. He had followed the advice of a breeder friend who said long-term Prednisolone would cause abortions and hurt the animal. He stopped the therapy.

The owner now agreed to follow the program faithfully and try again. We resumed the therapy. At the next cycle, the dog was bred and produced six beautiful puppies.

The moral of these stories is this: Side effects and long-term steroid therapy are not necessarily synonymous if you know what you are doing and are indeed treating a cortisol deficiency.

I don't suggest anyone use cortisone without first testing the patient's ability to produce cortisol. If the hormone is inadequate, replacement can restore balance. This method is precise. If used carefully, it does not cause side effects or problems. It resolves problems.

I believe the procedure I am suggesting can lay to rest the pervasive fear of indefinite steroids. Many of my patients are living safely — and with good health — on a lifelong prescription. The program gives many animals a good chance for recovery who might otherwise be doomed to suffer to be put to sleep.

From the safety standpoint you can monitor the cortisone periodically. Repeat the blood test. Recheck at yearly intervals or any time there might be a clinical development.

Check the estrogen and antibody levels. If the cortisone is properly administered, these markers should return to a normal range. Use these internal yardsticks to go along with surface appearances.

No one, I think, likes the idea of a cat or dog having to live on cortisone. But if you have a cortisol-deficient animal, you must use it. The animal may not be able to live well, or perhaps live at all, without it.

18

Prevention

Maintaining the optimal health of an animal and preventing disease means upgrading the attention and care you give it. Here are some guidelines to follow:

● Your animal needs the best possible food in order to enjoy the best possible health. Junk food — as with humans — will create junk health.

Read labels. Be alert to the slick language of pet food labels that camouflage garbage.

Stay away from by-products, chemical additives, high protein formulations and munchies loaded with sugar, salt and preservatives.

Ask your veterinarian for advise on the best possible food you can serve. Check out the health-oriented products in your favorite pet shop or health food store.

In Chapter Fourteen I explain how to prepare or purchase hypoallergenic food for your animals and how you can create a diet that will minimize or eliminate the common allergy problems suffered by many pets. Refer to that chapter.

● Supplement with minerals. Fortifying the diet in this manner can help keep your animal in the full bloom of health. See Chapters Six and Fifteen.

● To ensure maximum absorption of food and medication it's a good idea to have a simple and inexpensive enzyme test performed by your veterinarian. See Chapters Seven and Sixteen.

● Exercise is another important element in health. We know how important it is for us humans. And surely, in their natural environs, cats and dogs evolved on activity that was necessary for their survival. I recommend you contact your veterinarian for suggestions about how best to keep your animals in shape.

● If you think your animal has a problem, don't wait for it to get worse. Seek professional help.

● Keeping your animal clean and well-groomed is good prevention. Whether you routinely bathe and comb an animal yourself or have the job done by a grooming service, the close-up inspection involved offers opportunity to spot trouble before it gets serious. Such early detection can be a primary weapon against disease.

I have always felt that groomers in particular are in an ideal situation — working closely with animals, and often on a regular basis — to notice changes that may warrant veterinary attention.

I believe that keeping a look-out for irregularities should be part of the grooming routine, along with reporting observations and recommending professional treatment when necessary.

THE TEN-POINT HEALTH CHECK

I recently wrote an article for "Pet Age Magazine" in which I created a ten-point "health check" for groomers. The points can also be applied if you bathe and clean your animal yourself.

1. General impression. Take a general head-to-toe look. Is the animal limping, sluggish, hyperactive?

What's the general attitude of the pet? This is important because it can reflect how the animal is feeling.

2. On the grooming stand. Pet and caress the animal, making it comfortable. After all, it may not know why it is there and may be a bit uptight.

While petting the animal you can run your hand easily over the animal's body. Caress the head, the shoulders, the underside and backside. Basically you are looking for any bumps, lumps, tumors, warts, cysts. Anything out of the ordinary.

Enlarged mammary glands in a female can be a tip-off to pregnancy or a false pregnancy.

Secondly, you are making sure that when you start grooming the animal, you are not going to comb or cut into anything that might cause pain.

Does the animal look too thin or too fat? Either extreme can mean problems. When you run your hand over the animal body, does it feel thinner than last time? Weight loss is a common sign of disease.

3. Check out the coat. Stand back and view the entire hair coat. How is the coat for an animal of this breed? Is it nice and lustrous? How's the texture? Is it fine? Is it coarse?

Are there any areas of hair loss? This can often be a surface signal of a disorder inside.

What's the color? Are there any rust-colored stains? These could be signs of some disturbance, perhaps an allergy, where the animal aggressively licks or chews at his skin.

4. Perform a physical examination. Begin with the mouth. First, outside the mouth, look for any dermatitis, hair loss or abrasions near the lips.

Move inside and check the teeth. See if any are broken or coated with excess tartar.

Check the gums. Look at the gum line. If it appears red, this could indicate an infection, inflammation or buildup of tartar that should get some veterinary attention.

Pale gums may suggest anemia and, in the case of cats, announce the presence of the dreaded leukemia virus. In an older cat, pale gums can also be the sign of chronic kidney disease. Don't delay in seeing a veterinarian.

Look for any tumors or masses. Check the insides of the lips and under the tongue.

5. Check the ears. Lift the flaps. Look inside. Do you see any discharge? Is there a fetid smell inside the ears? A bad smell can signal an infection, excess production of ear wax, an allergy, or the presence of ear mites.

Is the ear flap thickened? Reddish, thickened tissue may mean there is an allergic reaction occurring, and perhaps an infection.

A reddish-blackish wax can be the sign of an ear mite problem. See your veterinarian soon.

6. The eyes. Check for overall clarity. Examine the iris, the round, pigmented membrane surrounding the pupil of the eye. Are there any film-like opacities covering this area?

Look at the whites. Is there any redness? That's a sign of possible inflammation and infection.

Look at the eyelids. Check for small growths, inflammations or styes that may be bothering the animal.

Is there excess spillage of tears from the eyes, leaving a rust-colored stain below. This can suggest an allergic problem.

7. The nose. Is there any discharge from the nostrils? This could indicate a possible allergy or infection.

Look for a loss of pigment on the nose. A black nose that turns pale could be perhaps a genetic defect or sign of a mineral deficiency. It might also be the result of the animal rubbing its nose excessively on one of those plastic feeding bowls every time it eats.

If the animal sneezes constantly and you find blood in the discharge, this can mean the presence of a a foreign body, such as a foxtail or piece of grass, or maybe even a tumor.

8. The rear end. When emptying the anal glands, check the color of the secretion. Brown is normal. A yellow or green color indicates infection.

Check the rectum area and tail for any growths. A bulge on either side of the rectum can be a perineal hernia.

Check for signs of tapeworms — small rice-like grains or balls around the rectum hairs. An animal with a thriving case of tapeworms will eat excessively to make up for what the worms are eating. The hair coat will be coarse. A potbelly is often present.

Moving to the genitalia, check for irregularities, inflammations. Observe the testicles to make sure there are no tumors developing...and to see that both are there. Some dogs are born with only one normally hanging testicle. The other is retained in the body. Studies have shown that tumors develop in 40 percent of undescended testicles.

9. The feet. Check the base of the nails for fungus or inflammations. Check between the toes for any foreign bodies, such as foxtails, or cysts that may be causing pain.

Look at the bottom of the pads for any cuts or punctures. Redness and inflammation on the bottom between the toes can be a sign of an infection, fungus, or a contact or food allergy. Any raw skin on the feet or up the sides of the legs can suggest excessive licking or chewing due to an allergic reaction.

If there are signs of licking on top of the paws — a rust-colored stain but normal, non-inflamed skin — this can indicate the possibility of poor circulation. Decreased blood flow can lead to tingling paws which an animal will repeatedly lick. A visit to a veterinarian is definitely in order here to determine if the animal suffers from a cardiovascular condition.

10. The skin. The animal is wet. You've just washed it. At this point, you can get a good look at the condition of the skin. You look for red, raw or raised areas, signs of a current inflammation due perhaps to allergy or infection. Patches of thickened or black skin can be signs of past problems.

THE RESPONSIBILITY OF BREEDERS

Breeders have a great responsibility for the future survival and health of pets. I am convinced that if current breeding trends continue — emphasizing a fashionable look and ignoring the health of breeding stock — cats and dogs may be bred out of popularity and perhaps out of existence.

Something has to change.

And that something is to elevate the health of an animal as the sine qua non of breeding practices.

An animal should be bred only after it can meet solid standards for health and vigor.

As long as breeders continue to worship at the shrine of glamour and relegate or ignore the health factor, a multiple injustice takes place — to the future litter, the future buyers and the future of the breed.

This kind of practice perpetuates unwellness, suffering and shoddy goods. It carries the seeds of genetic disaster for animals and financial ruin for the breeders themselves.

In the previous chapter I described how just one blood test can help determine the basic health of an animal. The test can be utilized both for curative and preventive measures.

I believe it offers an excellent opportunity to end the present allergy epidemic and health blight affecting millions of animals.

I believe it also offers an opportunity for the future — for producing viable animals, animals that are good and healthy as well as good looking. The indicators in this test can supply critical genetic data, providing the opportunity to withhold questionable animals from perpetuating disease and deformity.

I don't enjoy the sight of sobbing children carrying their grossly sick puppies and kittens into my clinic. I see too much of that: too many incurable animals, too many animals devastated by genetic timebombs, too many animals bred not for a long life but for an early death.

This situation is totally unacceptable and inexcusable.

I have tried in this book to express one veterinarian's view of a major problem and suggest how to deal with it. If the information presented here is not heeded I believe that Mother Nature will simply do the job herself — through continued crippling, sterility, early deaths, and eventual destruction of cats and dogs.

19

Is There A Human Connection?

The purpose of this book is to help animals. But might not some of the problems and suggestions I have raised also apply to humans?

Looking back at the many animals I have treated over the years with dietary and hormonal therapies, I have always wondered if we humans could perhaps benefit from such an approach.

When I see how epileptic dogs respond I think about the many people who suffer from this fearsome condition. They live lifetimes on anti-epileptic drugs.

Might they not be helped by looking into their diet for offensive foods and nutritional deficiencies?

Indeed, the field of nutritional medicine is making more and more correlations to health and the food we eat.

I find that many allergy conditions among pets respond dramatically to dietary and nutritional therapy. And here, too, physicians are linking many human allergic reactions to diet.

And what about the adrenal glands? In my clinical research, I have found that this tiny organ, and specifically a tiny secretion of a tiny part of it, to be involved intimately with overall health.

Does this also apply to humans?

Do we have genetically-flawed cortices from generations of eating adulterated food or glands damaged by a continual bombardment of modern-day environmental stress?

We have our eyes and hearts checked. But who ever gets his or her adrenals tested? I suggest that the crucial influence the adrenal hormones exert on the immune system makes a strong case for closer adrenal scrutiny.

I have come to regard allergies and many disease processes as "secondaries," that is, consequent to the adrenal problem. Perhaps some of the diseases of mankind are also "secondaries" to an adrenal weakness.

Might not some of the cancer, leukemia, the pancreas and liver diseases, the malabsorption problems, auto-immune diseases, and perhaps even AIDS, fall within the range of endocrine-immune imbalances?

I personally look forward to great revelations about health and disease as human medicine explores nutrition and endocrine-immune relationships. These two areas have yielded so much benefit to me and the animals I treat.

20

Pet Allergies Update

The response to this book, from breeders, pet owners and veterinarians alike, has been extremely gratifying. Since it was first published in 1986, many people have taken the time to call or write and tell me how they have successfully applied the recommendations I have put forward. From these unsolicited testimonials, it is clear that many, many animals who might otherwise have been put to sleep or destined to endure prolonged suffering have been helped.

I have continued to learn more about allergies and other health problems affecting our cats and dogs and in this update chapter I would like to share this information with you.

THE BREEDING CRISIS — FAINT GLIMMERS OF HOPE

Nearly five years after this book was written, the epidemic of improper breeding of cats and dogs continues unabated and the tragic fallout becomes even more intense. More than ever, I am seeing genetically-defective animals so damaged, so afflicted with complex problems, that they cannot be treated whatsoever. They can only be buried.

I have received SOS calls from all over the United States, from Canada, from Europe, Mexico and elsewhere. People are witnessing the same problems in various breeds of animals that I have been seeing in my clinical practice. The genetic timebomb is not restricted to Southern California or to the shores of the United States. It is pervasive — exploding and killing animals all over.

I and many other veterinarians are seeing Irish setters, Rottweilers, German Shepherds, Cocker Spaniels, Golden Retrievers, Shi-Tzus, Lapsa Apsas, Dobermans and other similar popular breeds being bred beyond the point of medical redemption. Among cats, the same can be said for Persians, Rex, Abyssinians, Himalayans, and Siamese. These animals come out miswired and malfunctioning — "designer" pets designed for death and suffering. They are born with bad hearts, defective immune systems, sebbhoreas, allergic dermatises, eosinophilic-gastroenteritises, and so on. There is no way to glue them together. You can only put them to sleep.

The sad part of this tragedy is that there is no coordinated effort to remedy the problem by strict controls at the breeding level. Still, we must all do whatever we can. We veterinarians can help by alerting the public through TV, radio and newspapers.

I hope concerned pet owners will be encouraged by this book to do the same. Sandy Wolfson, a client of mine, is one such example. She appeared with me on "The Geraldo Show" in the spring of 1990. Sandy had bought a Kairn Terrier from a prestigious New York City department store and thanks only to a most vigorous hormonal therapy and diet program, "Ardsley" is alive and healthy. The dog, now 8 years old, has multiple hormonal deficiencies requiring careful monitoring.

"Arnold," a second Kairn which Sandy had subsequently obtained, was beyond the best help I could provide, The animal had severe multiple deficiencies along with diabetes. After keeping him alive for five years, the timebomb exploded and we had to put him to sleep.

Both dogs were products of a Kansas puppy mill.

Whether we are considering the activities of factory-like puppy and kitten mills, backyard breeders, or the breeders of blue-ribbon champions, the inbred endproducts are equally defective. Lack of public awareness of the scope of the problem has enabled it to continue. That, hopefully, will change. Individual buyers must become aware that the problems they experience are not the exception, but the rule — one more example of a growing epidemic. Here in California, a state assemblyman has introduced legislation making it illegal for pet shops to sell unhealthy animals bought from puppy mills.

On the show level, ribbons and trophies should be disallowed as credentials for breeding unless an animal proves itself in its original design and function. That to me is a guarantee of health and stamina. We are starting to see that happen here in the United States as it has in England, France and Germany, where function tests are part of the championship competition for certain breeds.

Jack Russells, for instance, are now undergoing tough function trials in this country that put stamina, intelligence, obedience, sight and smell to the test. The winners are the hardy champions we want to breed, not the "Gucci Bags" that merely look good.

One day I would like to see a nationwide canine Olympics based on function. Those would be the dogs to breed!

Meanwhile, the blood test I have described in Chapter 17 is one tool we can use to ensure the preservation of durable animals. Roz Wheelock, a leading Southern California Doberman breeder, has used it with great success over the years to eliminate the health problems plaguing that breed. She has had beautiful puppies. Bill Shatner, who wrote the foreword to this book, recently purchased one of her Dobie pups. As a long-time aficionado of the breed, Bill noted that Roz's healthy pups were structurally larger and more solid than the run of contemporary Dobermans. This is how the breed looked originally when it was first introduced in America from Europe. Let's hope that the weak, wispy "designer" Doberman will give way to a big, strong, healthy, happy and born-again Doberman.

I invite my veterinarian colleagues to apply the research presented in this book as a powerful weapon against the current health epidemic. And I also urge them to generate or actively support efforts aimed at controlling puppy mills and tainted breeding practices. The time has come whereby the dollar cannot motivate the future of our pets. We have to take action and stop what amounts to genocide.

A WORD ON WHEAT

For many years I believed that wheat and wheat byproducts were highly allergenic to dogs. More recently, however, I have come to the conclusion that they are not as allergenic as I earlier believed and that in most cases wheat becomes a problem primarily when it is included in formulas with other food allergens.

You will often see wheat, wheat bran, wheat germ or wheat middlings used as ingredients in pet food formulas. These ingredients have the potential to add to the total allergenicity of the product when things such as beef, yeast and other foodstuffs listed in "hit list" (see page 20) are present.

I have had excellent therapeutic results over the years with a lamb and rice formulation that contains a good amount of whole wheat in it. Lamb and rice, in the vast majority of cases, are non-offending foods. Added to these hypoallergenic ingredients, the wheat causes no problems.

My recommendation remains to keep dogs off products with "hit list" foods. If you find a product that contains wheat without the other offending foods, your animal will probably be OK.

I have not found wheat to be a problem with cats.

GENERIC PRODUCTS

Buyer beware! Chances are that the cheap plain wrap pet food products sold widely throughout the country contain highly questionable ingredients. For years I have been concerned about these products and have recently learned that they are often reject or sub-standard chow sold out the "back door" by major manufacturers.

MORE ON MANGE

Over the years I had been puzzled by a number of cases in which I had put dogs on replacement therapy programs for hormonal-antibody imbalances and after seemingly thriving for a short period of time they would begin to develop pustular, scabby skin with open weeping sores. Generally, the therapy corrects skin conditions such as this. Blood tests showed their hormonal levels had indeed been normalized.

In time it became apparent we were dealing with an active, subclinical population of demodectic mange whose presence eluded even multiple skin scrappings. The eruptions were probably an allergic reaction to metabolic toxins produced by the mange as well as to defense chemicals produced by the host animal's own immune system.

Periodic baths with Mitoban resolve this problem. As the mange population is reduced, the skin clears up dramatically, usually within a couple of weeks.

Some animals require ongoing treatment with Mitoban — once a month or even once a week in some cases. I regard these cases as further examples of genetic damage where immune systems have been compromised to an extreme.

SELECTED REFERENCES

● Rowe and Rowe, "Food Allergy," Charles C. Thomas Publishers (Springfield), 1972.

● Alfred Plechner and Mark Shannon, "Canine Immune Complex Diseases," Modern Veterinary Practice, November 1976, p. 917.

● Plechner and Shannon, "Food-Induced Hypersensitivity," Modern Veterinary Practice, March 1977, p. 225.

● Plechner, "Food Mediated Disorders," California Veterinarian, June 1978.

● Plechner, Shannon, Arnold Epstein, Eli Goldstein, Edwin B. Howard, "Endocrine-Immune Surveillance," Pulse, June-July 1978.

● Plechner, "Theory of Endocrine Immune Surveillance," California Veterinarian, January 1979, p. 12.

● Plechner, "Preliminary Observations On Endocrine-Associated Immunodeficiencies In Dogs—A Clinician Explores The Relationship of Immunodeficiencies To Endocrinopathy," Modern Veterinary Practice, October 1979, p.811.

● Marshall Mandell and Lynne Waller Scanlon, "Dr. Mandell's 5-Day Allergy Relief System," Thomas Y. Crowell Publishers (New York), 1979.

● Wendell Belfield and Martin Zucker, "How To Have A Healthier Dog," Signet Books (New York), 1982.

● P.G.C. Bedford, "The Collie Eye Anomaly Problem," The Veterinary Annual, Scientechnica, Bristol (England), 1981, p.232.

● Plechner, "Feline Nutrition — Read the Label," Pet Age, November 1982, p. 12.

● Belfield and Zucker, "The Very Healthy Cat Book," McGraw-Hill (New York), 1983.

● Plechner, "Canine Nutrition," Pet Age, February 1983, p. 20.

● Dana H. Murphy, "Too Much Of A Good Thing: Protein And A Dog's Diet," International Journal For The Study Of Animal Problems, Vol. 4, No. 2, 1983, p. 101.

● R. A. Mugford, "Aggressive Behavior In The English Cocker Spaniel," The Veterinary Annual, Scientechnica, Bristol, 1984, p. 310.

● Plechner, "Skin Problems - Mineral Supplements May Be The Answer," Pet Age, November 1985, p. 24.

INDEX

Adrenal defects, 7-9, 35, 59-84,
    95-96, 106-119
Allergic HIT List, 20
Allergy, 5-6, 8-9, 25, 28-29,
    67, 85-91
  beef, 18-20, 29-30, 35-36, 39,
    75, 77
  corn, 21-22, 29
  eggs, 23
  flea-bite, 85-88, 113
  food, 8-9, 18-39, 44, 50-51,
    71-72, 75-78, 87-88
  inhalant, 90-91
  milk, 21, 29, 46, 50
  pork, 22-23
  tuna, 22, 36, 38
  turkey, 22-23
  wheat, 21-22, 29

Behavior, 33-34, 71, 74
Breeding practices and defects
    caused by, 5, 7-9, 52-68,
    123-124
Bronchitis, 35-36

Calcium, 46
Chemical additives, 14-17, 23,
    29-31, 120
Commercial pet food, 4, 11-17,
    28-32, 41-43, 45
Cortisol, 7, 60-85, 106-119
Cortisone [steroids], 7, 61, 65,
    80-82, 106-119

Ear infections, 71-72
Enzymes and enzyme deficien-
    cies, 6, 36-38, 48-51,
    104-105, 115, 117, 120
Epilepsy, 34-35, 75, 116
Estrogen, 63-65, 66 [chart], 75,
    89-90, 106-119

Feline Infectious Peritonitis [FIP],
    81-82, 112, 117
Feline Leukemia [FeLV], 79-81,
    111-112, 117-118
  vaccine, 81
Feline Urologic Syndrome [FUS],
    30, 38-39, 82-83, 112-113
Food byproducts, 13

Gastro-intestinal upset, 25-26,
    50-51, 71-72, 75-76
Gum disease, 78

Hypoallergenic diet, 6, 19,
    28, 33-38, 49, 71-72,
    88, 97-101

Immune system, 25-26, 31, 39,
    43, 60-67, 76, 89
Interdigital cysts, 27-28

Kidney disease, 14, 38-39

Liver disease, 36-37

Mange [demodex], 89-90,
    114-115
Medication impairment, 51,
    117-118
Minerals, 9, 40-47, 87, 102-103,
    120
Mites, 88-89
Mold, 23-24, 29

Pancreatic disease, 37-38

Reproductive disorders [females],
    115-116, 118-119

Salt, 15, 31
Skin disease [dermatitis], 26-28,
    31, 44-46, 50, 69-70, 72,
    83-84, 106
  flea-bite, 85-88, 113
  mange, 89-90, 114-115
  mites, 88-89
  inhalant allergies, 90-91
Sugar, 15, 31

Thyroid, 64, 66 [chart],
    109-111, 114

Upper respiratory disease, 84

Vitamins, 42
  B complex, 42, andfleas, 87
  vitamin C, 42

Yeast, 21, 29,
  and fleas, 87

Zinc, 40, 43-45